FAMILY LIVES AND HIDDEN SECRETS

THE BOOK THAT WILL SOLVE MANKIND'S UNANSWERED QUESTIONS ABOUT "LOVE" AND "HAVING CHILDREN"

KASEM KORBSRISATE, M.D.

Family Lives and Hidden Secrets

Published by KASEM KORBSRISATE, M.D.

First Edition

ISBN 978-616-577-227-3 (paperback)
ISBN 978-616-577-058-3 (ebook)

TRANSLATION: Nantavit Pornpibul
COPYEDITING: *WannaRite*
BOOK DESIGN: Phonthiwa Waiyakruttha

To

Pure and true love

in all children's hearts

Preface

Nature has created a large number of things. And to ensure that these creations will last forever, Nature has prepared certain mechanisms to control them. For instance, a variety of living things created along with the ecosystem for each of them, the Earth and other planets are held together in the solar system, and families can be viewed as a system for humans as well. We're so familiar with these things that we think no mechanisms are playing their roles behind the scenes.

This book will discuss family lives because they're so close to us and play a very important role in bringing happiness into our lives. Learning about the rules and mechanisms of family lives is particularly vital. However, this masterpiece of Nature is so delicate and complicated, it's not easy to explain and to cover all facts involved.

If there are mistakes or flaws found in this book, I'm willing to be fully responsible. And if you have advice or suggestions, feel free to contact me via the following channels:

- kasemkasem007
- korbsrisate@gmail.com
- https://www.facebook.com/kasemkorbsrisate

Lastly, I hope this book will benefit the general public by offers a better understanding of family lives and helps strengthen family institutions in order to bring happiness to mankind as long as possible. That's the way Nature intended.

Kasem Korbsrisate, M.D.

Contents

Having Children: A Coincidence or Nature's Intent?

How Does Nature Motivate Us to Have Children?

Married Couples with Children and Positive Changes

Having Children: A Coincidence or Nature's Intent?

Introduction

Why Did I Write This Book?

Can We Trust Our Feelings?

Why Do We Have Children?

Why Did I Write This Book?

When my first child was born, I was around 43 already. At the time I had quite a lot of life experiences even though my lifestyle was not so exciting or adventurous. As a doctor, I spent most of my time in hospitals and rarely traveled upcountry. However, I still came across unfortunate or life-threatening events. For example, I almost drowned twice on boat trips and lost more than 10 friends and teachers in a boating accident. I've witnessed countless different types of deceptions in our society, many of which ended with violence such as murder.

Therefore, I think it's a good idea to share these experiences with my children and younger generations so that they would be cautious and prepared. I'm so motivated that I wrote 6 books altogether and this one you're reading is the 6th. Originally, my plan was to publish all 6 books. But the situation of the publishing industry has changed to the point where even major magazines and newspapers were forced to close down. After much thought, I decided to publish only this book instead since its content is deeper and more interesting than the rest. The main purpose of this book is to help you "lead a happy life."

This topic is so important because when we graduate, our lives will no longer be limited to "studying, playing (after school), and taking exams." Some of us will be free for at least 8 hours on workdays for several decades. The period after graduation until death takes almost or more than half of a person's life. Those who enjoy their personal lives will find the world a wonderful place to be. As for those who don't, the older they get, the lonelier they will become. And this is not a favorable situation.

Lifestyles can be categorized in many ways. But if we look carefully, there are 2 main types:

1) Living single: Eating, drinking, traveling, and enjoying all kinds of recreational activities available to choose from
2) Starting a family: Getting married and having children

Since making the right choices affects our lives tremendously, we should carefully choose our lifestyle based on as much information as possible. And this is why I wrote this book, the book that will help you choose your lifestyle more wisely.

Can We Trust Our Feelings?

Naturally, our feelings tend to lead us to think that we're always right and others are wrong. For example:

- If we ask people who use European cars, e.g., Benz and BMW, why they chose to buy them, they will tell you so many good things about these cars. But if we ask those who use Japanese cars, the answers will be totally different.
- The rich are likely to feel pity for the poor; they're lacking financially, cannot travel, and have to lead difficult lives. On the contrary, the poor also feel pity for the rich; they spend all their time making money but do not have time to use it, to enjoy the beauty of lives, and to be with their families; their beautiful houses are there mostly for their housekeepers to enjoy.

Similarly, if we ask a single person whether it's better to stay single or get married, the person will tend to bombard us with reasons to stay single and problems caused by getting married. On the other hand, if you ask a married person, you will get completely different answers. This will definitely cause a headache and confusion to anyone who tries to ask such a question because they won't know who to believe. Feelings naturally make us have bias towards ourselves or see only the world on our side (our own world), which is not necessarily a bad thing. In a way, it helps us feel at ease and brings about a peaceful society because everyone is satisfied with his/her situation.

To decide whether to stay single or get married cannot be based solely on someone else's opinion. It's crucial to think deeply and logically about consequences in order to come to the right conclusion for each of us. Therefore, this book will describe each factor in detail so the readers can make informed decisions when the time comes.

A few things I should be clear about before discussing my ideas:

- The content in this book can be used to help you make a decision. I have no intention to bluff or claim that one way is better than the other.
- Building a family is not a simple thing. There are a number of obstacles. Understanding reasons for having children and details of family lives encourages one to overcome these obstacles. However, building a family will be successful or not still depends on numerous factors.
- Even though starting a family is a good thing, it should be done at an appropriate timing to prevent some problems. For example, a couple should wait 3 - 5 years after graduation or until they are over 25 years old to be mature enough. Waiting for the right time also helps build a stronger foundation for a family.

Why Do We Have Children?

Nowadays, people have much better general knowledge than before. We're more knowledgeable about both trivial and important matters such as the origin of the universe and global warming. Although some affect us very little, we've learned so much about them in detail. For instance:

- How many megapixels do the front and rear cameras of a new model of that smartphone have? And what are the new features?
- What can a smartwatch do? When will they launch a new model? And how will it be better than the previous ones?
- In how many years will autonomous cars be available?
- How far has the space tourism project gone?

What I've mentioned above affects our lives very little, yet we seem to know lots of details about them. On the contrary, some issues have significant impacts on us but we understand them very superficially.

One of these issues is **"reasons to have children"** or **"how having children change our lives."**

In the past, not knowing why we have children didn't lead to any problems because other options were not available. Humans didn't have any other sources of happiness apart from their families. Therefore, when they became adults, they would want to have loving families and beautiful children. They would take this route without having to know other additional details.

However, nowadays we're no longer in that situation. We've abundant sources of happiness to choose from. Owning just a smartphone with a Wi-Fi signal can bring limitless joy and excitement. Thus, a large number of people spend day and night looking at the screens of their phones. That is why we call this phenomenon "a phubbing society" which has spread throughout the world.

If reasons to have children are not clearly revealed in detail, this way of life that has brought happiness to mankind for hundreds of thousand years will be overlooked or even ignored. These days we're surrounded by numerous forms of entertainment. Advertisement billboards around each intersection, messages sent to your smartphones or on the Internet, and brochures handed to you offer all kinds of entertainment products. When we get distracted like this, we gradually lose interest in building loving families.

Thus, it is crucial that this book explains the facts of family lives that are still missing so that the readers can have a different view which plays a vital role in the happiness of mankind. These facts will also help you choose an appropriate lifestyle.

Nature and Living Things

Advantages of Assumptions

Laws of Nature and Overlooked Facts

Advantages of Assumptions

Family lives are complicated and involve many different kinds of hidden mechanisms, so understanding these facts is not easy. One way to help us understand difficult matters more easily is by "making an assumption." Assumptions have been used in different fields of sciences, especially physics:

- A molecule is the smallest fundamental unit of a substance that can exist independently. A molecule consists of a group of atoms bonded together.
- Molecules of every substance have the strength of electrostatic attraction among them. Attraction among molecules of the solid is stronger than those of the liquid. Therefore, the solid doesn't change its form to fit its container.

No one has seen molecules or atoms; however, science accepts that both exist. This is because assumptions can be used to explain natural phenomena accurately. And since assumptions help us understand difficult issues more easily, two assumptions that will be used to explore family lives in this book are as follows:

Assumption 1: Everything that we call "nature" such as sea, sky, or living things including humans, has been meticulously created. They were designed and planned very carefully in advance. This is not different from masterpieces found in different professions, e.g., tailors, film directors, painters, and novelists, whose works consist of numerous complicated steps. Thus, in creating these masterpieces, they had to plan and implement these plans delicately step by step in order to achieve perfect outcomes.

I made this assumption due to the fact that every system in nature like the universe, ecology, and human body, (e.g., digestive system and respiratory system) is so complicated it's hard to believe that this is due to evolution, trial and error, or coincidence. On the contrary, they must have been meticulously planned. And the builder/planner must have known about these systems deeply to achieve such level of success.

Assumption 2: Nature could not cause these creations to happen easily, so there must be a system set up to ensure that they will exist forever. And if they were ceased to exist, recreating them might not be possible. Furthermore, these systems are interdependent. Extinction of one system such as the disappearance of trees, sea, or insects, will inevitably have a drastic domino effect on other systems.

These two assumptions are not complex, they are so simple and logical it's not difficult to accept. As for who "the creator" is, although we don't really know, there are various words for the creator like "God" or some prefer to use "Nature." Thus, many people believe that "God" and "Nature" are, in fact, the same thing. As for the issues regarding:

- Who is the creator?
- Are God and Nature the same thing?
- Does God really exist?

They are rather complicated; it should take another book to explain these issues. Besides, no matter who planned these systems, the two assumptions: "they were meticulously built" and "once completed, they have to be maintained to last forever," are still valid.

And since I don't know who the creator is, I use the word "God" or "Nature" depending on the context. I don't know if God really exists but I sense that the word "God" has a deeper implication, is easier to understand, and more concrete. So I use these terms interchangeably.

Laws of Nature and Overlooked Facts

In order for her creations to last forever, Nature prepares certain mechanisms for living things such as plants and animals so that they keep breeding continuously:

- Hens with the ability to lay eggs and give birth to chickens which will eventually become hens capable of laying more eggs
- Trees with the ability to bear fruits, allowing them to breed unceasingly

Nature creates different kinds of laws to support these processes, ensuring they are carried out smoothly. For example, to make animals feel the urge to breed and to make mothers love and take care of their children. However, these laws have certain interesting characteristics:

They are not 100% accurate. As for "Mothers will always love and protect their children," we know that it's not always the case.

Some animals eat their own children and some cats simply walk away without feeding their kittens. Although there are many cases like these, the abovementioned law is still true. In fact, no rules in the world are 100 percent accurate, as the saying goes, "There is an exception to every rule." Sometimes certain factors interfere in ways that cause the outcomes to vary one way or another.

Some laws are more flexible than others. For example, alcohol and cigarettes go against the law of nature that "our bodies need fresh air and healthy food." But we can drink and smoke for quite a while until abnormalities start to surface. And even when the abnormalities have emerged, people who want to go against nature (by drinking or smoking) could still continue these habits. Abnormalities and diseases are simply signals reminding them that these habits are not good for them and should be given up, otherwise their bodies will stop functioning. These signals act like speed bumps on the road, they only give a warning that drivers should slow down but some drivers would still continue speeding up even though their cars may break down.

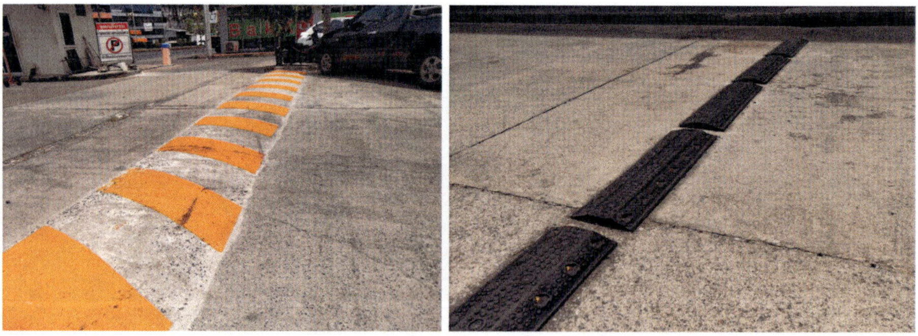

| Speed bumps

Some laws will function only at appropriate timing. Several innate mechanisms will only function at appropriate timing. This can be clearly seen in the case of lysosomes.

Each cell has lysosomes. And each lysosome contains hydrolytic enzymes that can break down the cell and itself. That's why they are also called "suicide bags" or "suicide sacs," they can destroy everything around them including themselves.

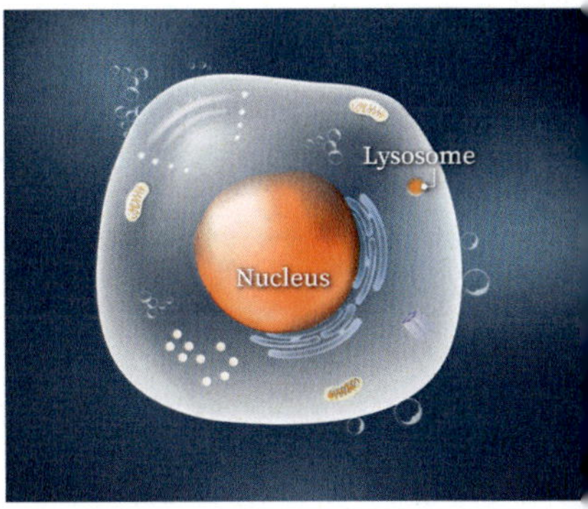

| Lysosome

In other words, animal cells always carry bombs with themselves and will explode at appropriate timing.

- When an animal dies, lysosomes will start to digest their cells, resulting in decay of their bodies.
- When tadpoles turn into frogs. Lysosomes digest their tails.

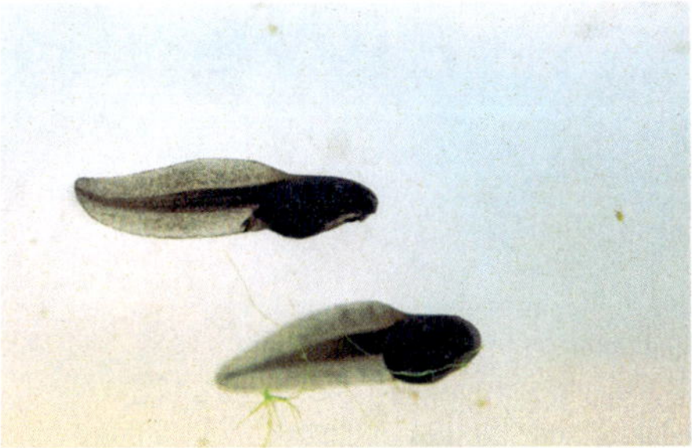
| Tadpoles

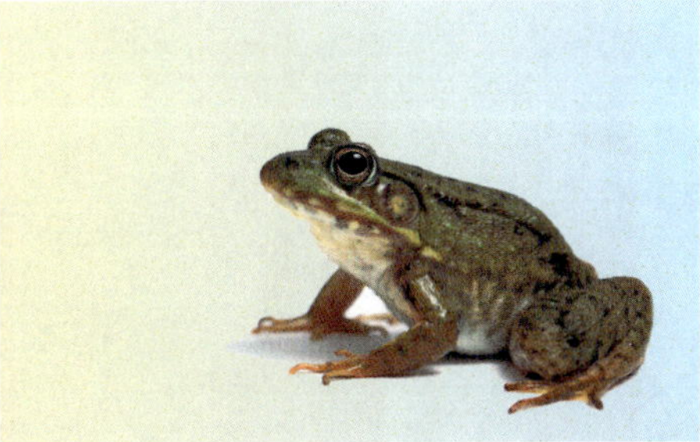
| Frog

The long tail of a tadpole disappears when it has become a frog. Lysosomes play a role in digesting its tail. Although lysosomes already existed in its cells for quite a long time, they won't start functioning (by digesting the tail or themselves) unless it's time to do so.

Similarly, Nature has also built several other mechanisms hidden in our bodies that stay inactive until the appropriate time arrives. The role of lysosomes is to help humans continue to exist for a very long time. In the chapters that follow, I will discuss these mechanisms in detail.

Mechanisms That Create Love

Love Between Young Couples

Love Between Parents and Children

Love Between Young Couples

Although Nature wants living things including humans to continue to exist, it is essential that their numbers must not be too high. Whether their numbers are too high or too low, there will be negative consequences on the balance of nature. Therefore, Nature uses "matching" as a mechanism to control these numbers. That is, most kinds of animals on earth can breed only after matching with one of its opposite sex. Most cannot just breed by themselves. This approach cuts down the increasing rates to half because it takes 2 animals that successfully match to produce their young. This controls not only their numbers but also selects the fittest animals to breed. That is, the female will choose the strongest and the most capable male to breed with. Weak and unhealthy ones are less likely to be selected. Through this "matching," Nature can control both the quantity and quality of animals on earth simultaneously.

What Nature uses to ensure that "matching" will happen is "love," in which lust and sexual desire play a part. Matching begins when we become teenagers, the age where there are a number of mental and physical changes. Also, there are some behavioral changes. For example, teenagers prefer spending time with their friends to their parents. These changes go on until there is a new kind of emotion in their heart, "young love."

This kind of love is different from love for their parents and friends because it is full of passion and hidden energy. People in love can behave unexpectedly:

- They can starve to the point where they become so skinny or on the verge of fainting just to be admired by their lovers that they're in better shape.
- If their love happens to be interfered, some are willing to sacrifice everything, e.g., work, their parents, friends, and education, just to be able to spend their lives with their lovers.
- If they're deceived by their lovers, love may turn into rage. Some committed suicide or killed those who cheated on them.

Love between a couple is so strong because Nature knows very well that most of these young people still live in happy homes with their parents who are taking good care of them. Separating them from their parents and urging them to get married are no easy tasks. Thus, Nature has to find a new technique to take them away from the lifestyle they have been comfortable with. Similarly, gardeners use fire or heat to force the bees out of their cozy nests. Therefore, Nature designed love between young couples to be as passionate and intense as a fire burning. Those who are at the stage where they're madly in love with someone tend to be impatient and restless. They only want to go out to see their lovers instead of staying at home. Therefore, there are several love metaphors used with the words related to "fire." For instance, one's heart on fire; one's latest flame; getting burned.

However, sometimes the heat or hidden energy of love results in negative consequences. Some people were so heartbroken they committed suicide or killed those who caused their love to end. This is because they might have prior psychological problems such as depression or a tendency to have strong feelings. Without these psychological problems, sadness due to being heartbroken is not likely to be so severe and lasts around 3 months. It will gradually disappear and when they've found new lovers, they will be joyful again. Thus, heartbroken people should take good care of themselves for at least 3 months until the sadness fades away and things will slowly get back to normal.

The overall picture suggests that young love plays an important role and carries with its strong passion, otherwise "matching" will not occur and humans would not be able to sustain their species up until the present time.

Love Between Parents and Children

When we talk about love, most people always think of love between young couples. Movies and songs often mention love between young lovers. Rarely do they talk about love between parents and children. People tend to overlook this type of love and think there is no point to talk about it.

The climax of each movie that we've seen often shows a couple who plays the leading roles get married "and live happily ever after." The entertainment industry gives us the impression that getting married is the most valuable thing and nothing else after that is as important. But in reality, Nature has prepared many other scenes waiting for us to take part in because, for Nature, the objective or the climax is not "a marriage" but "sustaining human species," in other words, "giving birth to children."

And to guide us to head towards that stage, Nature sets up "a mechanism of happiness" to welcome those willing to step into the path towards "having children." At the same time, she builds mechanisms that work like speed bumps to slow us down, to cause problems or irritations for those who choose not to go in the direction she has provided. These mechanisms are placed and hidden neatly throughout our lives. Only those who observe will see them.

What Nature has prepared to welcome these people is "happiness from becoming parents." But this form of happiness will occur only when both parents and children genuinely love each other. Nature knows well that the more they love each other, the stronger the happiness they would gain. Thus, Nature designs a new kind of love for them — the deep and firm one.

This masterpiece of Nature is not only exquisite but also complicated, it's not easy to explain. This book is rather longer than others since I have to proceed slowly. Several things are unexpected or even beyond ones' imagination. So, the readers must read carefully. Whatever way you choose to read this book, at the end you will understand family lives much better than before.

How Love Develops

The Loveliest Child in the World

Creation of Love Between Mother and Child

Toughest Hazing

Warnings for Love Building

The Loveliest Child in the World

Due to the fact that Nature wants all animals including humans to produce their young to sustain their species, she has prepared love and happiness as rewards, otherwise no one will want to have children. And humans would not be able to sustain their species for hundreds of thousand years.

To elaborate on this matter, let me discuss a proverb in a calendar I received in 2012. The calendar contains a collection of sayings and proverbs about the love between mothers and their children from different countries, one of which is a Chinese proverb translated into English:

"There is only one prettiest child in the world and every mother has it."

Proverbs are often facts of lives that have been overlooked. They have been written down to remind people or to emphasize the importance of these facts. After reading this proverb, many may not understand why there is only one prettiest child in the world and why every mother has that child. This is because Nature has provided a mechanism that makes every mother thinks in the same direction: "My child is the loveliest one." And when she thinks that way, she feels that she owns the loveliest child in the world just as the proverb described. This phenomenon occurs with every child in each family. And it has nothing to do with the physical beauty of these children.

To help you understand this more clearly, please take a look at these lovely children.

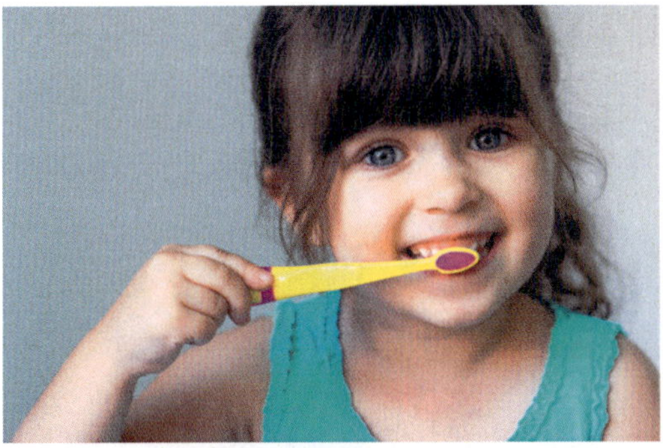
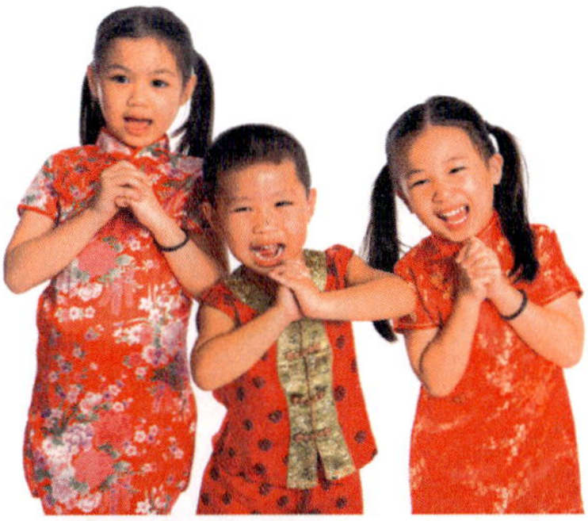
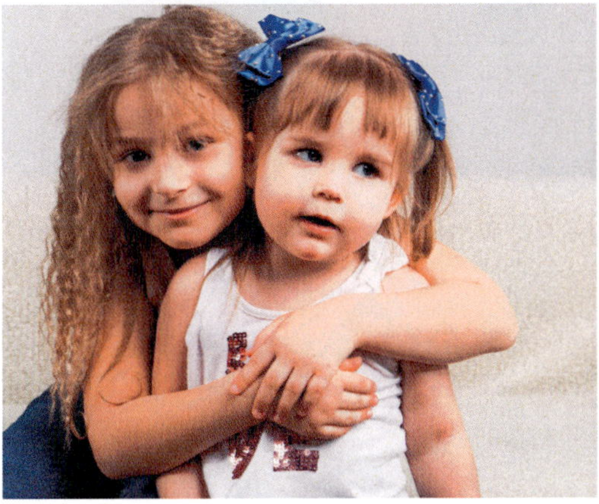
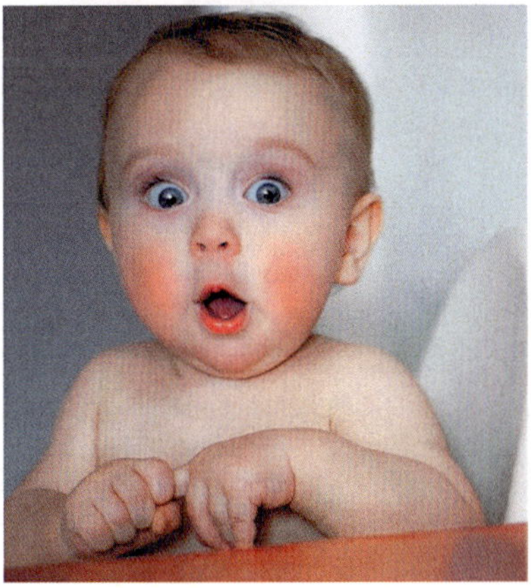

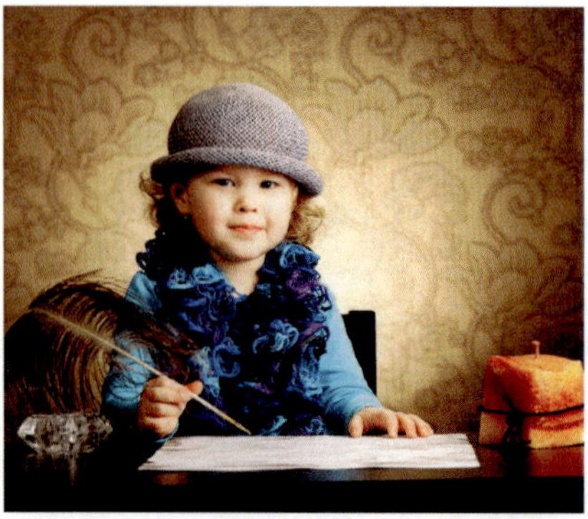

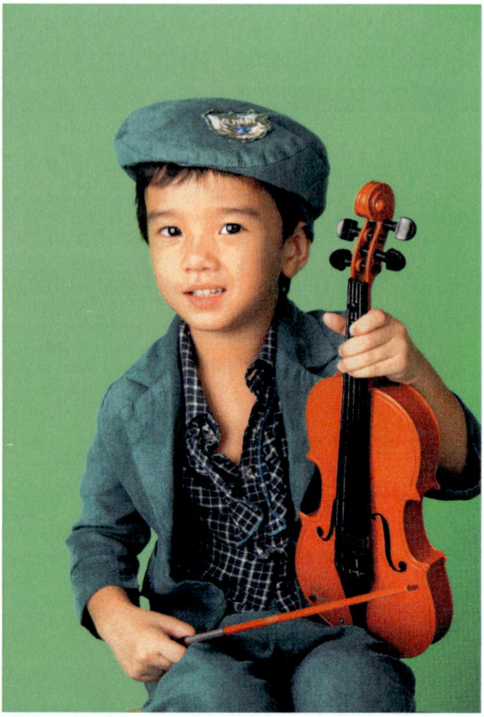

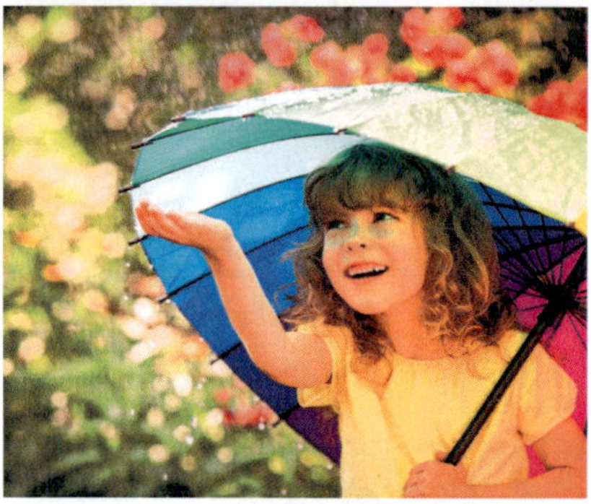

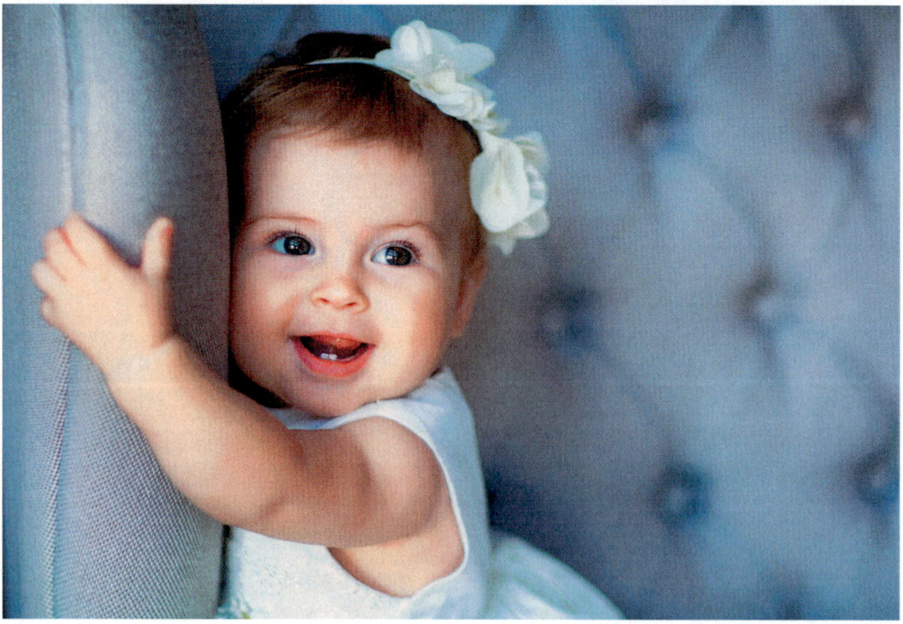

People in general make decisions about a kid's appearance from what they see. That is, if the kid is good-looking, they would say this kid is "lovely." But a mother makes a decision based on the mother-child connection. It has nothing to do with the kid's appearance. This bond is so strong and genuine from the bottom of their hearts. Therefore, it is worth more than what can be seen from outside. No matter how beautiful the children in these photos are, these children cannot be as beautiful as theirs.

Naturally, the mother-child connection and the feeling that she's with the loveliest child in the world bring a great deal of joy and pride to the mother. This is normal for anyone who owns the most precious and beautiful thing, or in this case, the loveliest child in the world. This kind of happiness makes the time they spend together, which may last as long as 20 - 40 years, a series of happy moments.

Neither appearances nor disabilities can change the fact in this proverb. For example, when a child was born without limbs or with brain damage, a mother's feeling remains unchanged. She still feels that "My child is the loveliest one in the world." Thus, every mother enjoys happy moments with her child or children no matter what problems may arise. This is in accordance with Nature's intent to reward all mothers with happiness based on love. Poverty or richness; beauty or ugliness, any form of abnormalities can never take away this great and pure maternal love.

Creation of Love Between Mother and Child

Because dangers are all around, Nature creates love between mothers and their babies to shield them from all kinds of dangers. Without maternal love, they may not be able to survive. That means the extinction of all species including humans.

This type of love is quite different from other types, so the mechanism that creates it is also different. As for young love, Nature utilizes changes in their bodies, i.e., hormones and sexual desire as the main drive to create this type of love. But as for the love between a mother and her child, Nature uses "exhaustion and troubles" to bring it out.

The main principle is that "when two people choose to live together and to go through obstacles and troubles in their lives, they will start to bond spiritually." And this kind of love can be felt only within the hearts of those who have experienced a series of tragedies together. People who didn't go through these situations cannot feel the love that gradually emerged.

This fact is observed and used widely in "a hazing"[1] in educational institutions. If the activities involved are used properly and do not put freshmen's lives at risk, they can be very useful in uniting people in a short period. Without these activities, it may take years for this to happen. Some students may attend the same classes for 2 - 3 years but never talk to each other. But "a properly planned hazing" can bring them close together quite quickly within only one day. After the hazing ends, they may joyfully tease each other or call their new friends by their nicknames.

Only one day can create such a strong bond. When Nature puts a mother and her child together in similar situations continuously for years, how much will they love each other? It's not surprising all mothers feel the same way that "their children are the loveliest kids in the world." Nature intentionally creates the strongest bond between them. Furthermore, each mother also feels that "My child is the most precious thing in the world." Next, I will discuss ideas regarding hazing activities in detail.

1 "A hazing" involves activities organized by university students, mostly sophomores, to welcome freshmen in order to adjust their behaviors and create unity. Usually, there are games and competitions that stress and exhaust participants.

Toughest Hazing

The tougher the hazing, the stronger the love and connection among people involved. However, if the hazing was organized by people who are not knowledgeable enough, freshmen's lives may be at risk. They may die or become disabled. For example, some sophomores may force freshmen to drink several liters of water. Eventually, this may accidentally kill them by causing a sudden cardiac arrest or kidney failure although they didn't have any prior diseases. So, the organizers have to be particularly careful because if things go wrong, they may be put behind bars instead of staying in a university. On the contrary, Nature doesn't have the same problem because she understands all the systems in human's body very well before creating humans. A hazing designed by Nature may seem tough but actually, it is safe. Rituals involved aim at creating a bond between a mother and her child. The highest point of this kind of bond is that she can literally "die in her child's place." Such a sacrifice can also be found among soldiers who have gone through a series of troubles together and developed a bond strong enough to risk their lives to help their buddies who are being surrounded by their enemies. They're willing to risk their lives although they are just friends. Because having to struggle through tough training together has created a strong bond and unity among them. This kind of love is the strongest and it's what Nature wants to ensure that the child, or her descendant, will be cared for and protected from dangers in the best way possible.

Suffering can unite people, it's the heart of hazing rituals or taking care of children. If you've met "a mother/father with an infant," or whoever is caring for a newborn baby, you will notice that the person looks pretty much the same, getting thinner and having tired eyes. In other words, they look like zombies. And they often say something like "Looking after a baby is so tiring." or "Why is raising a child so exhausting?" This is because taking care of an infant is a tough job. There are so many activities involved they cannot rest properly. Therefore, their physical health starts to decline. Some of the activities are:

- Giving the baby formula or breastfeeding every 2 hours and placing it on your shoulder or patting on its back. Putting the baby down right after feeding will cause it to throw up.
- Getting the baby to go to sleep when it starts to cry out of sleepiness, singing a lullaby and rocking the cradle or doing other things. Sometimes it takes as long as half an hour. It can be said that "an infant cannot fall asleep by itself." Without being lulled to sleep, a baby may cry for an hour.
- If the baby has a fever, the caregiver has to rub its body with wet cloth to lower the temperature. Without taking this action, it may have a seizure. Even at 2 or 3 a.m., the caregiver has to get up to do this because only a fever medicine may not be effective enough.

The parents can take care of their personal matters such as eating and taking a shower only when the child is asleep. Things will go on this way day and night even on weekends or public holidays. That's why the parents look so exhausted. If they are lucky, this will last only 6 months because the kid will start to sleep longer. That is, the baby will wake up every 4 hours instead of 2 hours to feed. The caregiver will have more time to rest. If not, they will have to wake up every 2 hours for 1 - 2 years until the baby starts to sleep longer. Not only is caring for a child as tough as hazing rituals, but it is also quite similar to participating in sports day organized for unity among school children.

Preparing formula. An infant wakes up to feed every 2 hours both day and night. The formula has to be freshly prepared. If the baby wakes up to feed 3 times per night, the formula has to be prepared 3 times. In order to prevent the child from suffering from hunger, it has to be done as quickly as possible because the baby will cry so loudly. This is quite similar to the game "filling up a bottle" shown in the picture:

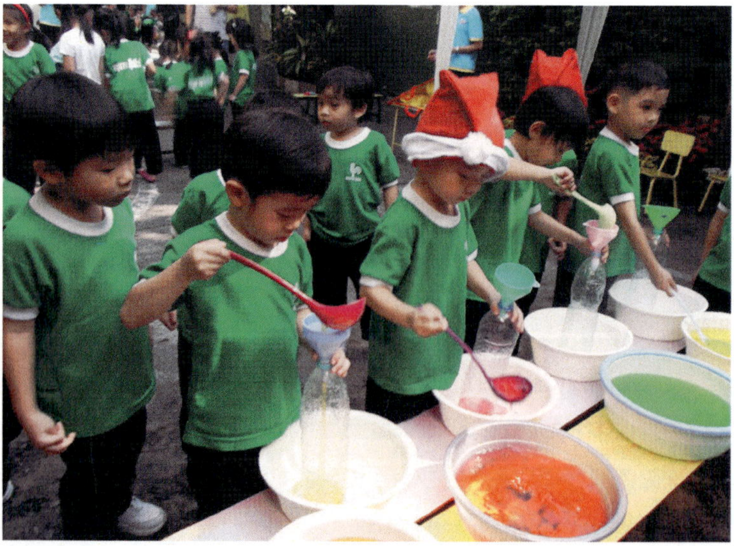

| a game called "filling up a bottle" (Photo from Klubpetsuksa School, Songkhla Province, Thailand.)

However, mixing the formula is much tougher than "filling up a bottle" because:

- It's "a game" that lasts 24 hours per day. And the worst part is the game will also go on during 2 - 4 a.m. when the parents are likely to be woken up from a deep sleep by a very loud cry of the child. This is like firefighters who are sleeping tightly, and when the siren goes off, they have to jump up suddenly. They cannot just dilly-dally.
- It's a good idea to add just a little bit of hot water to make the formula warm. So, this seems more like a game called "filling up a bottle *with hot water.*" And if the person is very sleepy, the hot water may spill on him/her quite easily.

Receiving vomit. Babies throw up very often when they're sick. After coughing violently a couple of times, they may also throw up. As shown in the next illustration, the parents have to prepare a tray to receive the vomit so that it will not mess up the bedsheet.

Receiving a child's vomit must be precise and quick. And parents cannot choose when to play this game even during 3 - 4 a.m. When they hear the child coughing, they have to be ready instantly. Importantly, they must not miss it. The person may hold the tray in his/her right hand and use the left hand to hold the baby. Gently pat the child's back if possible. If the caregiver had missed it, vomit would spill all over the place. So, this task requires good concentration and precision the same way children play "receiving a ball with a basket."

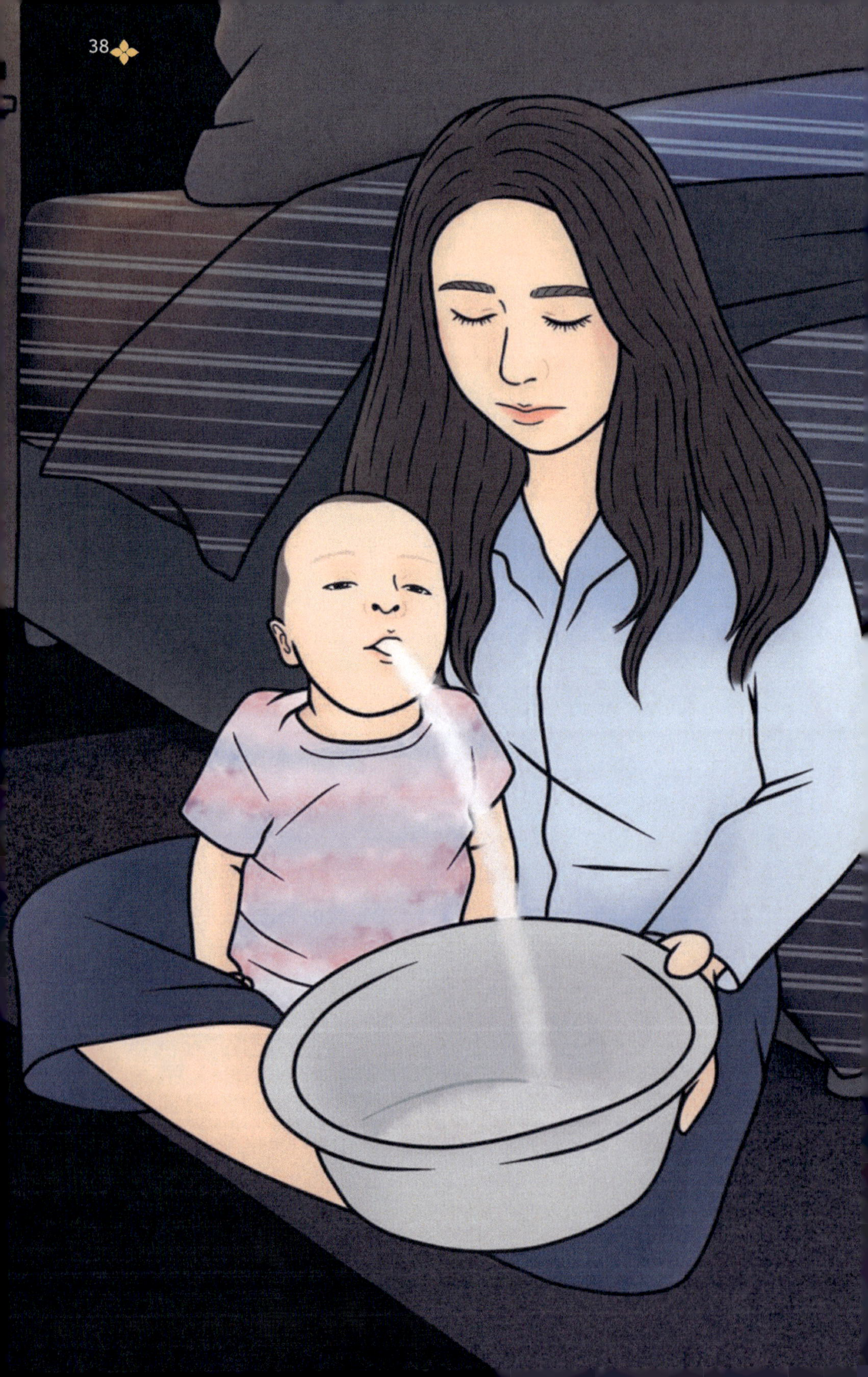

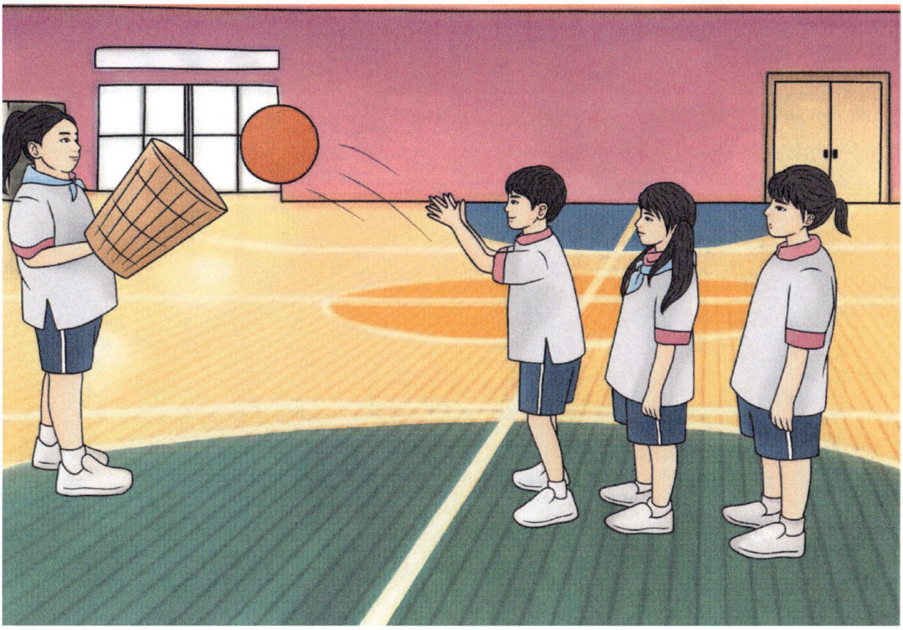

Each thrower tries to throw the ball into the basket. While the basket holder tries to receive the ball. The team that can receive more balls is the winner. (For kindergarten or elementary school kids, this is already quite difficult.)

Don't forget that at the time the room may be so dark you can barely see anything. The child is likely to be crying and uncooperative, its head is probably moving from side to side just like a fire fighting nozzle. So, it'll be very easy to miss. Besides, if you miss only once, the vomit will spill all over the bedsheet, pillowcases, and clothes. Everything will have to be changed at once. And it might be 4 or 5 a.m. when you're really sleepy. Sometimes you think the child has stopped vomiting, so you leave the room to clean the tray in the bathroom. But once you return, the bedsheet and the blanket are covered with vomit because the baby threw up while you were away.

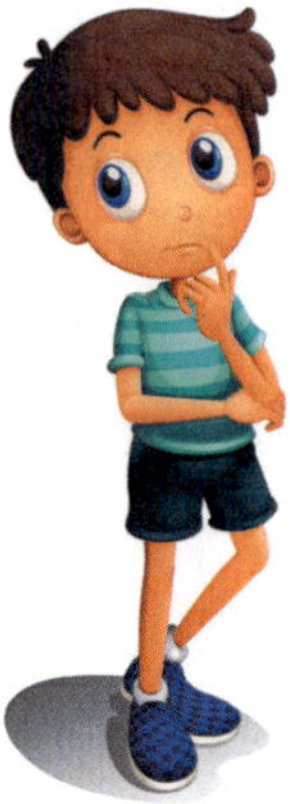

So, it must have been quite convenient for mothers who breastfeed their babies or caregivers before the time of baby formula because they wouldn't have to prepare the formula or play sports day games. Right?

This is not true. I compare caregivers' tasks to sports day games to let you see how exhaustion and troubles help develop the kind of love among people involved. Taking care of infants has never been an easy job. It has always been a great responsibility. This is why the bond between mothers and her children has always been strong in all ages. What's more, this mechanism is dynamic. It can be more or less active. For example, some children were born with disabilities or fall ill quite often. Their mothers have to care for them more closely. The more they care for their babies, the more exhausted they become. And the more exhausted they are, the stronger the bond. As a result, the love that has increased gradually will give these children a chance to survive.

Warnings for Love Building

There are some matters about love-building mechanisms that should be understood:

It takes longer than 10 years to develop. Other kinds of animals depend on their mothers for not so long. Some species can take care of themselves after a few days. The kinds that spend more time with their mothers take only a few years. Nature forces mothers to take care of their young until they are ready to survive by themselves. For humans, it's usually more than 10 years. Thus, this duty requires a deeper type of love, not just a superficial one, otherwise they will simply walk away from their young ones due to boredom. Forming a deep bond within every mother is not a simple task. To achieve this, it takes knowledge of thoughts and emotions. But for Nature, this is not a problem at all because she understands humans thoroughly. She can develop this kind of love easily through an unusually long period of ordeal so that love developed through these troubles and exhaustion can be absorbed slowly into mothers' thoughts. This is not different from letting the sauce slowly and thoroughly seep into a piece of meat. Or when you want to ensure that the deepest part of a big chunk of chicken is well cooked, you need to take more time. Similarly, mothers have to be submerged in troubles and exhaustion long enough for love to be absorbed by all parts of their thoughts until they think their children are the most precious gifts in the world and they will never abandon them no matter what problems may arise. This fact is apparent in many disasters such as an earthquake, a house on fire, and a sinking ship. We've seen deeply moved pictures where dead mothers holding their children, because even in the worst situation, a mother will not leave her child behind, she'll be willing to die there beside her young one.

It is necessary to take part fully in the game. Love is a result of going through obstacles and troubles together, therefore, we must participate fully in these situations. Others cannot play those roles for us. For example, we cannot let someone else join a hazing for us and hope that people at the university will like us when they know almost nothing about us. The best time a bond and love will develop is the nighttime because it's our normal bedtime. The activities during the nighttime cause more exhaustion and stress. Therefore, even millionaires with a great amount of money have to play this game by themselves, no one else can do it for them. Others may lend a hand occasionally or in case of an emergency.

Love based on this approach is more valuable and plays a greater role than blood ties. You may have heard about babies from 2 families being swapped at birth by accident. Their parents did not realize this until almost 20 years have passed. They wondered why they didn't look or act like them. After a DNA test, they realized that the person they had been taken care of for more than 10 years didn't share their DNA. So, they started searching for their real child. After they met him, the mother felt he was like a stranger to her. Even when he was standing right in front of her, they didn't feel any connection. In the end, both families decided to sue the hospital that made a mistake and chose to continue raising the same children who were not really their own.

Taking care of infants is very exhausting. Therefore, a bond developed during this period is particularly firm. This tie makes the next 20 - 40 years full of joy and happiness. Thus, although during this period the parents may always look exhausted, the outcome is worthy. This is similar to receiving a vaccine injection which usually results in a sore arm. Still, it's worth the pain because you'll become immune to a disease for a long period. That's why we should enter this period with patience and a proper understanding that invaluable happiness is on its way.

What Love Brings to Family

Connection Between Parents and Children

World's Greatest Comedians

Mysterious Smiles

After this specific kind of love
has been established,
there will be other mechanisms
that follow to help family lives
to continue smoothly:

Connection Between Parents and Children

When parents have developed a connection with their children to a certain point, they will start to feel their children's happiness or sadness within their own hearts, for example:

- When a child laughs joyfully, the parents will also feel happy.
- When a child cries sadly or when he/she's in pain, the parents will suffer too.

The degree of happiness or sadness of the parents is almost exactly the same as their children. Whatever feelings the children experience, their parents will share those feelings. This is so similar to 2 electronic devices connected via Bluetooth that makes the main device and the connected device function as though they were one singular device. In the case of parents and children, it's their love and bond that connects their feelings.

However, before this kind of connection emerges, there must be some kind of parings during the period when the parents were taking care of their infants because the bond would be strongest during that time. Parents who didn't look after their own infants are not likely to gain this kind of paring. But if the pairing is complete, this parents-children connection will be established and bring about some changes in the parents:

- Even when the parents become as old as 70 - 80 years of age and can barely walk, they can still feel joy at a swimming pool or a tennis court because when their children are having fun swimming or playing, the happiness is also transferred to them.
- A convenience store near their house will turn into an amusing shopping center. In the past, only going to big malls or shopping abroad would bring that kind of joy, but when they have small children, even a small convenience store on a roadside can bring happiness the same way a big mall can. To small children, all kinds of goods are usually new and bring excitement to them,

> e.g., cheap toys or old CDs from 30 years ago. They would be so excited and happy if they can get them. So, they find these small convenience stores so entertaining. When the children are happy, so do the parents.

Happiness does not necessarily originate from the parents themselves anymore. It may be transferred from their children. Most parents can sense this form of mechanism, so they look for a source of joy for their children more often than for themselves. They prioritize their children, knowing that the happiness of their children will eventually be transferred to them. Those children who can easily find joy in their lives will make their parents happy easily as well.

Happiness induced by this mechanism appears every day and many times per day. These parents are fulfilled. They don't feel the need to travel abroad to be joyful the way they did in the past because a wonderful source of happiness is already in their own homes. Although it's the kind of happiness they gain easily without having to pay for it, it comes with quality. Nature knows well that raising a child is an exhausting task, so this form of happiness is "a gift from Nature" for these parents, the kind that melts stress away and turns child-rearing into fun activities. Such happiness that brings laughter and joy to the parents is so important when combined with some facts that I'm going to describe.

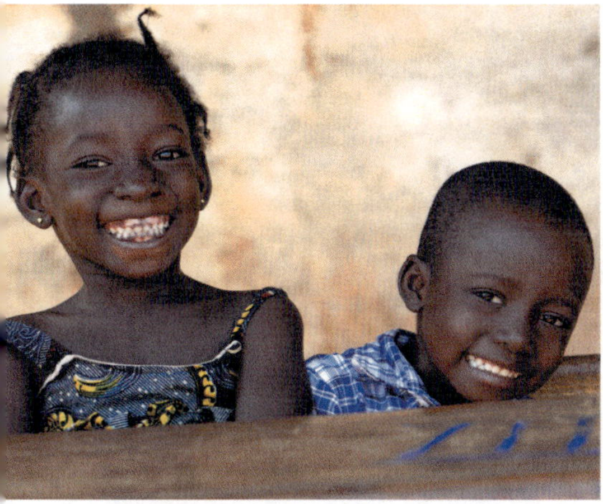

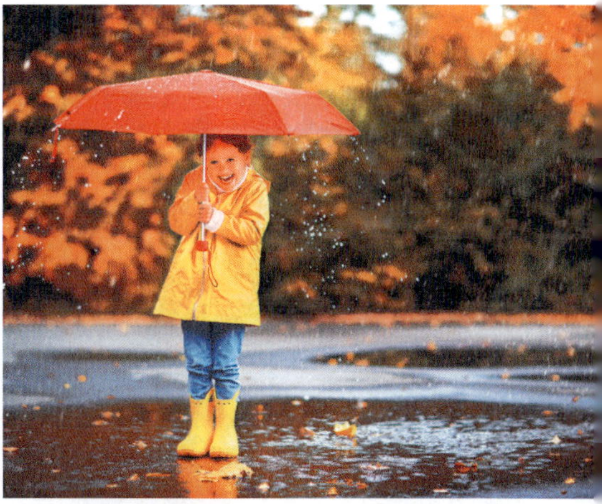

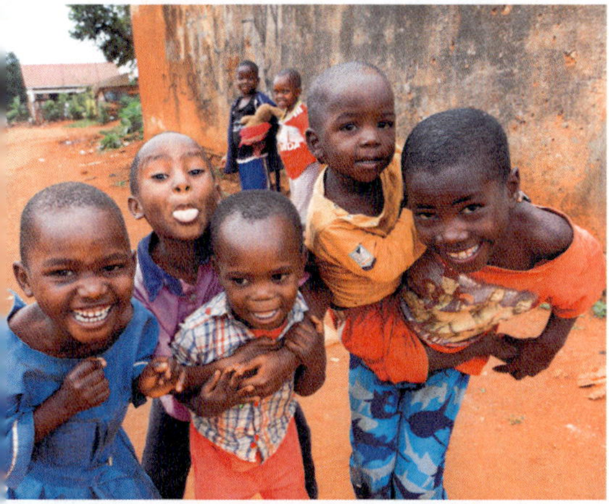

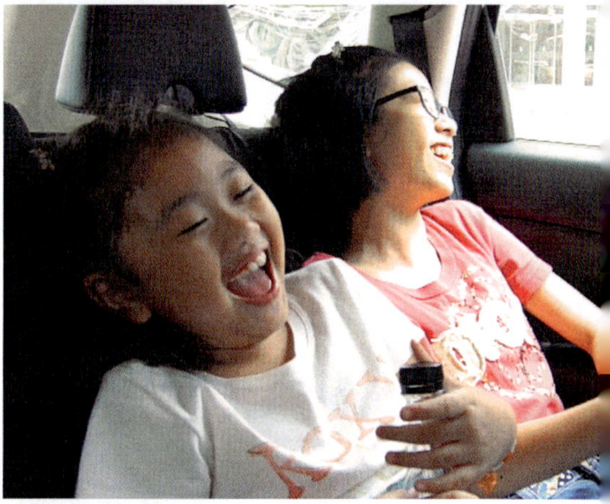

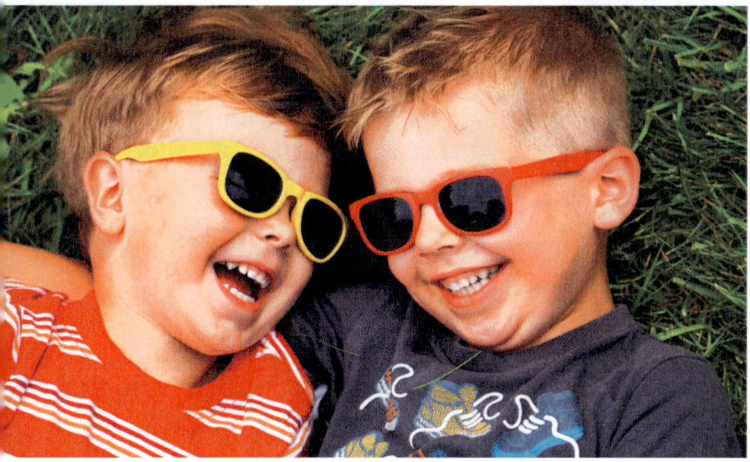

Children laughing (It's incredible but true that children naturally laugh about anything. When they laugh, the parents can also feel joy and amusement.)

World's Greatest Comedians

Before discussing the content of this part, there are 2 facts that you should know:

1. We cannot always trust our feelings. Some are accurate; others are not, as seen in the following examples:

- If you put your right hand in hot water and left hand in cold water. Then put both hands in room temperature water. Each will feel the opposite although it's in the same bowl of water.
- A superb dish from a fancy restaurant may be blamed for being too salty, too hot and spicy, or too sour. But for some people, food made by themselves may taste "quite good," "just about right," or "even better than those from a restaurant."
- When our kids quarrel with other kids. We are likely to think that our children are on the right side although we may be wrong.

Therefore, a feeling and a fact may not necessarily be the same thing.

2. We don't have a device capable of measuring people's feelings. Thus, we use one feeling to measure another. That's why each person tends to receive a different outcome. For example, a dish tastes "good" when it was made by yourself, but when others try it, they may disagree. In such a case, we tend to bias.

Similarly, a bond and love, after firmly established, will make the parents think about their children positively. For instance, they tend to think that their kids are smarter or prettier than other children. And when their kids talk about something slightly funny, they may think it's hilarious.

Case 1 A 7-year-old girl called Nalin went for lunch with her mother at a food court. While they were having lunch, they saw an old lady, aged around 70, walking toward them with a walking stick in one hand and her other hand is on a table to support herself while walking.

Nalin : Mom, what's wrong with her?
Mother : Oh. She's old. It's hard for her to walk around.
Nalin : If it's hard for her to walk, why doesn't she run instead?
Mother : ???

Case 2 At some point, news about children being abducted was the talk of the town. So a mother taught her boy to be more cautious about strangers.

Mother: Son, if a stranger approaches you or comes out of nowhere to talk to you, just run away. OK?

Son: OK, Mom. But uhmm, should I run to the right or the left?

Both cases may sound slightly funny to people in general. But for their parents, it was enough to make them rock with laughter. Children's behaviors can cause their parents to feel overjoyed or more satisfied than usual the same way food made by yourself is more delicious than how it actually tastes. Thus, for the parents, their children are the greatest comedians in the world.

Children make the house seem like an amusement park. They're like jokers who are a source of endless jokes. When the house is filled with laughter, exhausting activities of raising a child prove to bring joy and happiness. That is, Nature's intent to make child-rearing a source of happiness eventually becomes reality.

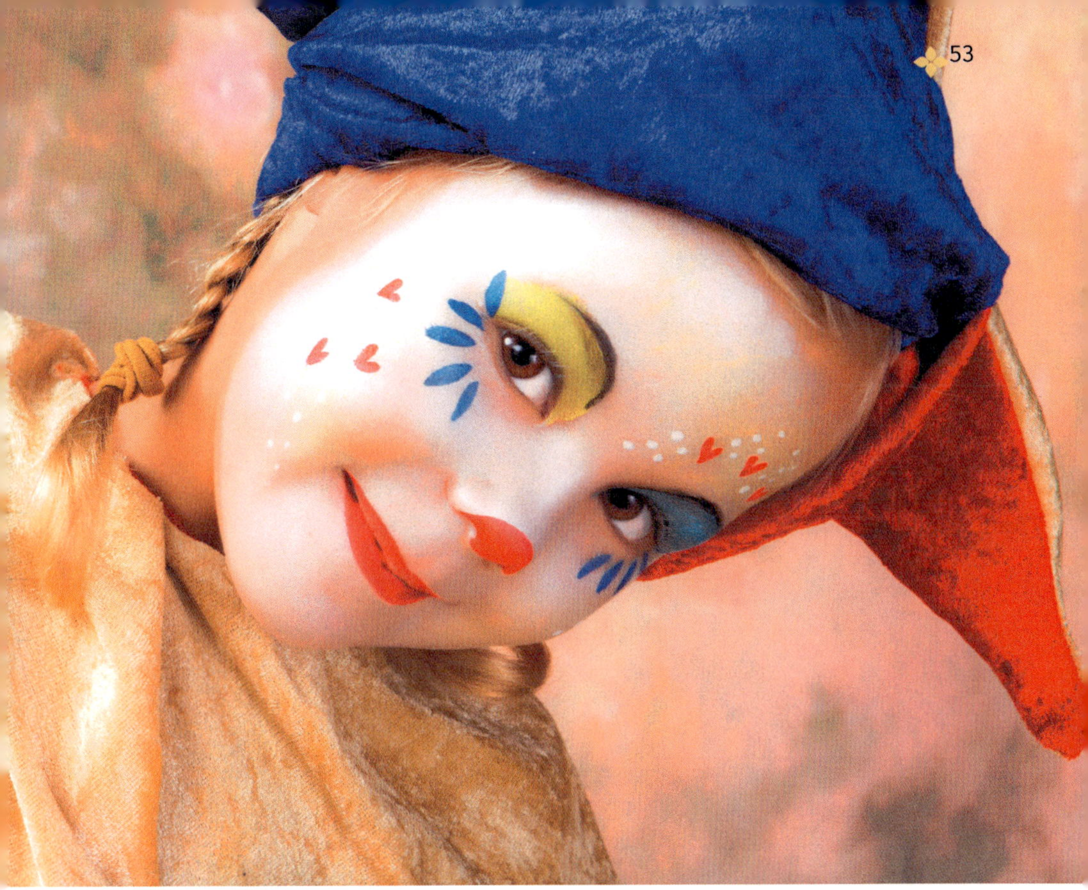

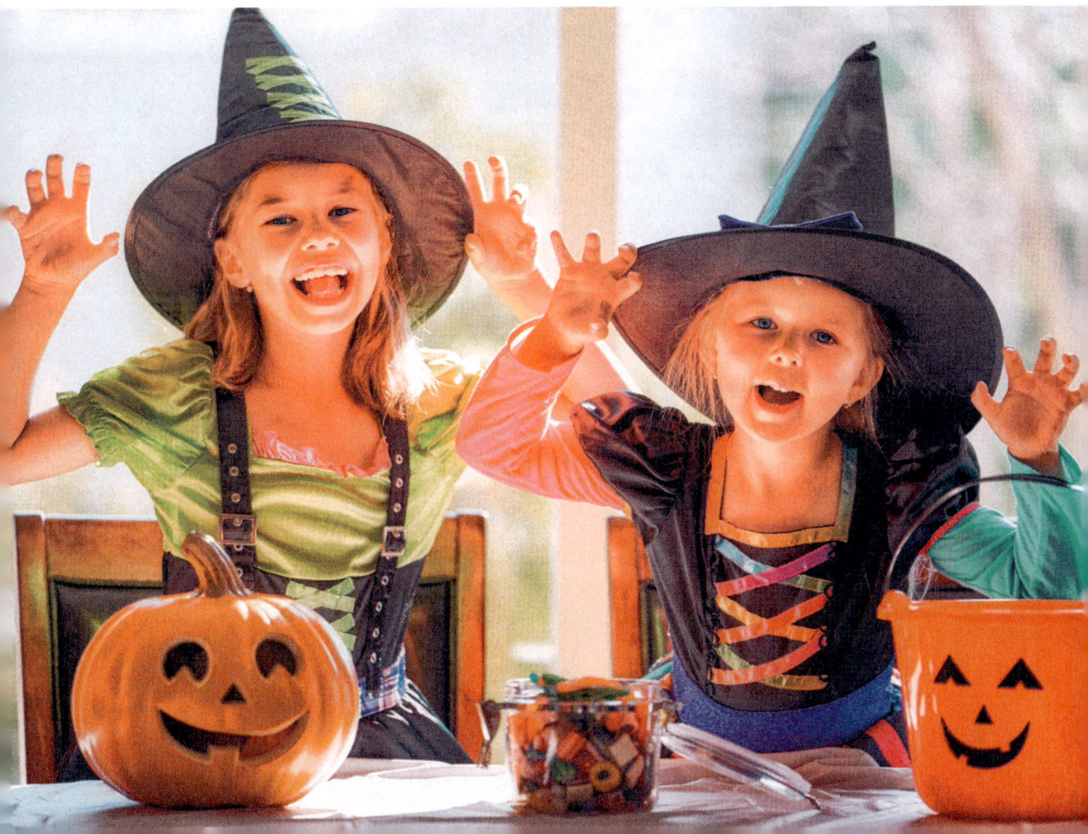

Mysterious Smiles

Many people have heard about the painting called Mona Lisa which is well-known worldwide. The artist, Leonardo da Vinci, created this masterpiece over 500 years ago.

The painting is not only beautiful but also mysterious. There are several theories regarding this painting, including Mona Lisa's "mysterious smile." A number of analysts tried to search for a message behind it. It seems like she's hiding something.

But there is another kind of smile that is also intriguing. It has a unique identity and keeps some hidden messages similar to that of Mona Lisa. You can see such smiles in the pictures:

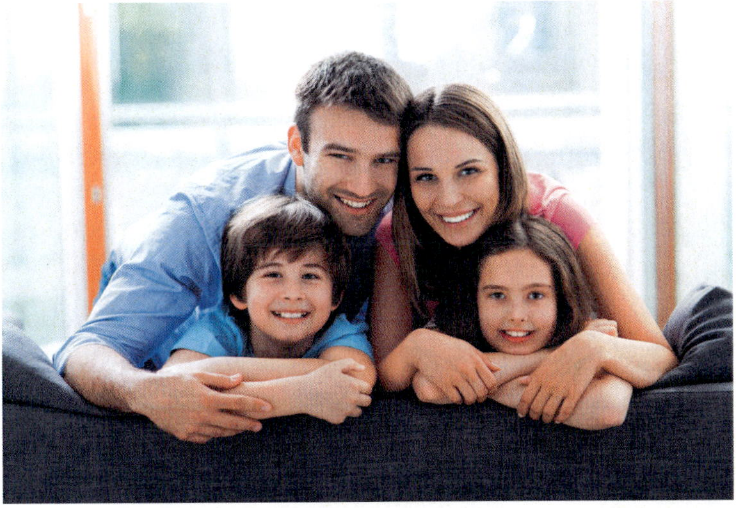

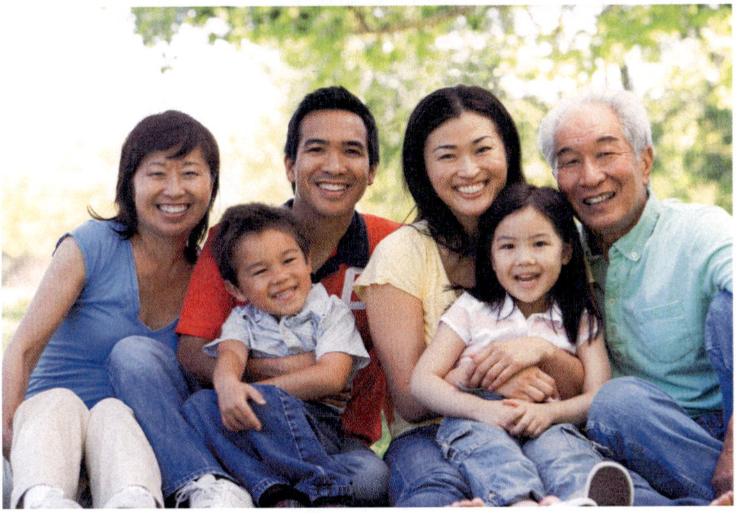

| Pictures of family lives

You may see that these people give a bigger smile than usual. It almost seems like they were laughing. But actually, they are just smiling. We may call this unique smile "a half-laugh-half-smile." This can only be seen in happy families. And it's different from the kind of smile when you're with friends or boy/girlfriend. When you're among friends, you tend to laugh. And when you're with your boy/girlfriend, you often smile slightly, not as wide and sincere as this.

In general, we smile because we're satisfied with something. How your smile will look, e.g., wide or narrow; awkward or willing, depends on various factors like moods, stress, and happiness/sadness during the time. Smiling is the sum of all feelings within one's heart:

- People who are nervous often give an awkward smile.
- Although orphans who have received a monetary donation or new school uniforms will smile gladly, their smiles reflect sadness because they're dealing with several problems such as families, education, and money to buy food.

We can learn a lot about people from their smiles. People give "a half-laugh-half-smile" because they are also happy about other things on top of what they're smiling about. This kind of happiness is special and can be found only in family lives. It's called "warmth in the family." How much this kind of warmth brings happiness can be seen in the facial expression of the lioness and her cub in the picture below:

| A lioness and her cub

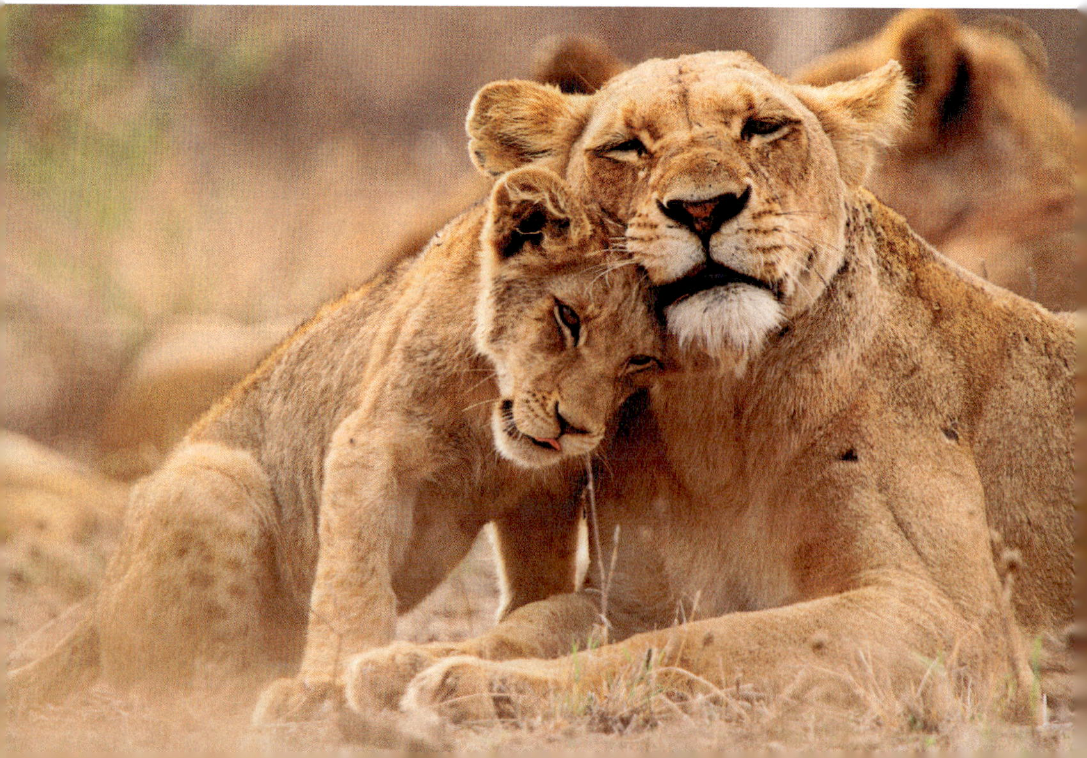

Happiness in families with children is unique. It's a sum of several kinds of happiness combined:

- Happiness from children transferred to their parents, (similar to 2 devices synced via Bluetooth).
- Happiness from the greatest comedians in the world who perform free of charge several shows per day.
- Happiness from warmth in the family just like the lioness and her cub. The more family members, the merrier.

When people are happier than usual, they smile more widely. This is an identity of family lives. These mysterious smiles are the key to the hidden secret that "Within a simple family life, there is a special kind of happiness." Thus, it's not surprising that former generations usually urged their children to get married and have children of their own. They knew wholeheartedly that their kids would naturally find this special kind of happiness the way they have experienced before. And they want their loved ones to feel the same thing.

Why Is Happiness in Family So Special?

Available Daily

The Best Life Drive

A Gift From God or Nature

The Main Element of Happiness

One Way or Another,
We Struggle for Happiness

Happiness based on love and warmth in a family is unique for the following reasons:

Available Daily

Stress occurs daily. We shouldn't let it build up and cause problems in our lives. So, we must find a way to eliminate it regularly the same way garbage on the street needs to be cleared daily to ensure that the city is clean and tidy. Otherwise, there will be a number of problems, e.g., an outbreak of flies, rats, and diseases. Similarly, there are other things we should get rid of daily to keep our mind balanced such as:

- Hunger
- Sleepiness

Owing to the fact that hunger and sleepiness are inevitable, we cannot eat or sleep only on certain days. But we have to eat and sleep every day to be healthy and to avoid health problems. Likewise, stress needs to be eliminated daily or it will accumulate in our brains like a rope tangled together to the point where it is hard to come undone. Releasing one's stress is similar to unfastening a tangled knot before it causes a big problem and other kinds of damage.

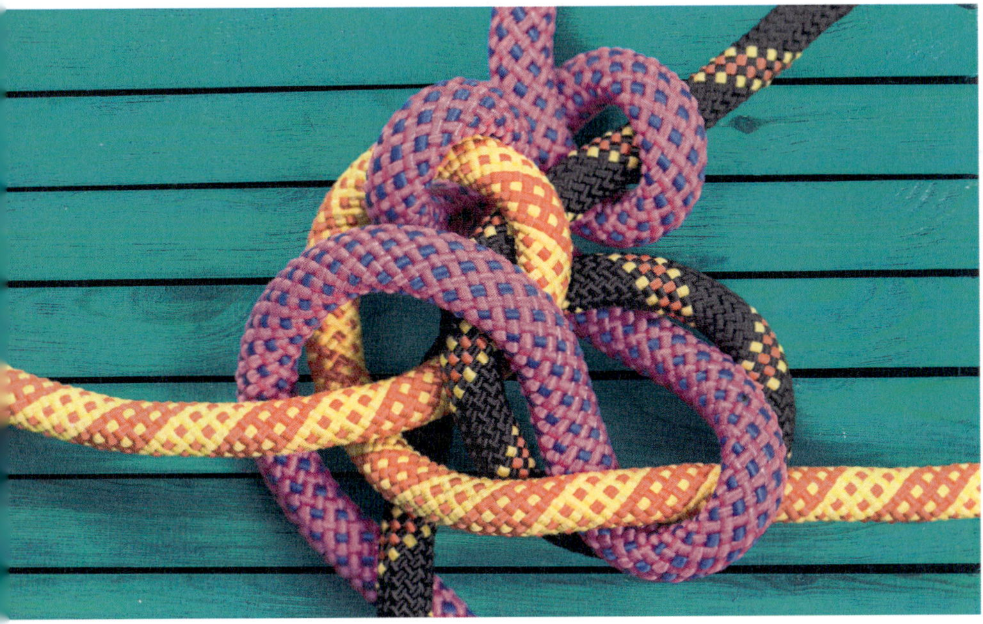

| Tangled Ropes

People release their stress in many ways:

- Some prefer exercising.
- Some enjoy traveling domestically or abroad.
- Others like going shopping, listening to music, or going to a movie.

That is, activities capable of making you happy can naturally melt down your stress. And raising a child is a source of happiness, so it can release your stress as well. Moreover, happiness from child-rearing has other characteristics.

Happiness parents can enjoy every day: The process that brings about this kind of happiness occurs at home, there is no need to step outside. You simply stay at home and wait for the entertainment to begin. Furthermore, its effect is instant. Once the parents return home from work and step inside the house, their children will run toward them and yell out "Dad!" "Mom!" Suddenly, their exhaustion just melts away. When compared to other kinds of happiness like traveling abroad, they are quite different. You possibly have to wait for at least three months to enjoy one trip. This means there are three months for stress to accumulate before it can be released, which is definitely bad for your mental health.

Happiness that is constantly changing its forms: Some might say they've plenty of money, they can go abroad whenever they want. But do you realize that the same kind of happiness that occurs repeatedly will eventually be no longer effective and stops bringing happiness? This is why people endlessly searching for different tourist attractions and shopping places to go to. And this is not a simple task because a new place has to be better, more luxurious, or more exciting than the previous ones to bring the same degree of happiness. The mechanisms behind this kind of happiness are exoticism and excitement. Even though you can afford to travel every week, it doesn't mean that you'll definitely be happy. If there is nothing new and exciting, you'll just feel indifferent. This is similar to people who go to international conferences regularly. They may get bored and probably prefer taking a rest at home.

However, happiness in a family comes from a child whose behaviors are developed in relation to their ages. A child is like the same hardware with its parts and programs being upgraded all the time, his/her appearances (hardware), thoughts and intelligence (software and CPU) gradually changed. The same child may act so differently as if he/she was a different person while growing up. His/her role as a joker has changed as well. It seems as though you keep having a new joker to entertain your family. But it doesn't end there. This kind of happiness comes from a bond and love among family members. The longer we live together, the stronger the bond. And the stronger the bond, the happier we are. Thus, it's less likely that such happiness will become ineffective like other kinds of happiness.

Happiness with a precious outcome: Don't forget that "child-rearing" is "a job," not "an entertaining activity." Nature is the one who makes it entertaining. And since it is a job, it brings an outcome. That's why raising a child is totally different from other means of seeking happiness. Other activities, e.g., going to a movie, listening to music, traveling, diving, or other fun activities bring you only entertainment. When time has passed by, what's left may be memories, photos, or video clips. But as for child-rearing, the result is "a person" who can love their parents in return. This is what we call "gratitude." You can see some examples in the photos below:

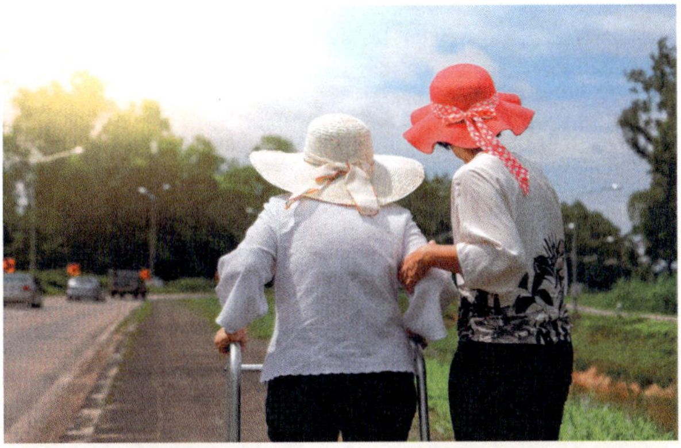

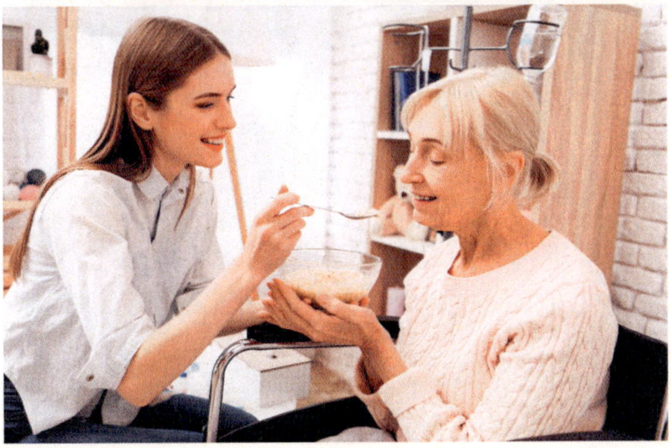

Apparently, the time you spend on child-rearing will not be wasted. This is because raising a child is full of laughter and the love dedicated to the child is kept in his/her heart just like saving money. When the parents get older, children will turn all the love saved in their hearts which is abstract into something concrete to contribute to the wellbeing of their parents.

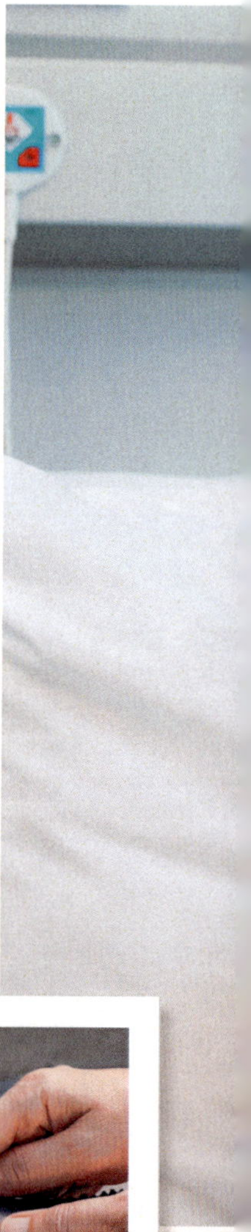

As a result, it's incredible that happiness in a family can change its form to match the parents' needs. From the time a child was born, the family is filled with laughter. A child had made home feel like an amusement park for decades. Even when the parents grow old, their children can still bring happiness to their lives. And it's the only kind of happiness the parents want. This is because, for the elderly, a million-dollar supercar, the latest model of a smartphone, a 10-carat diamond ring, or other valuables cannot bring joy to their lives. All they want is love and warmth from their children. These are what they use to fight against all kinds of diseases and life crises in their twilight years.

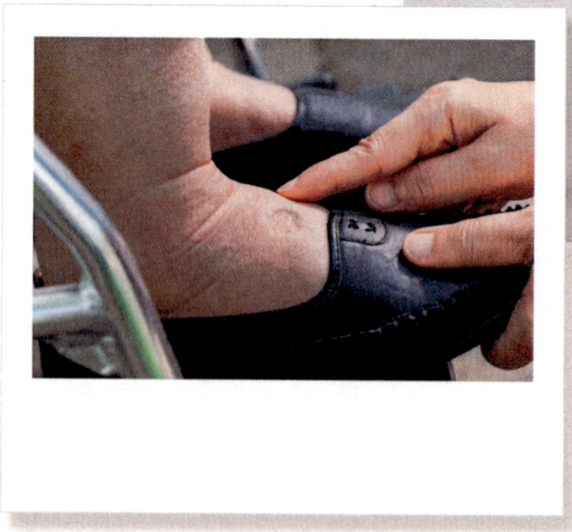

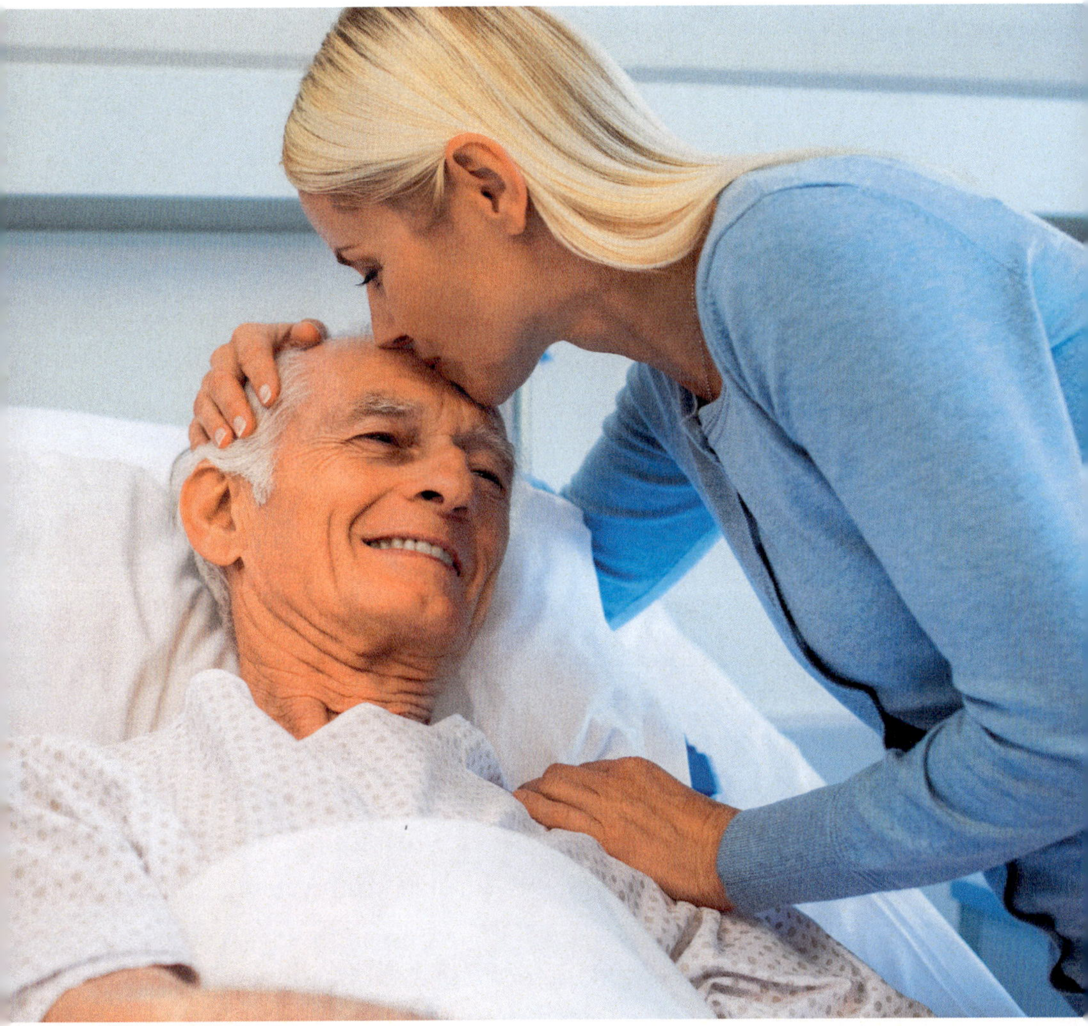

The Best Life Drive

Nature encourages humans to sustain their species by filling family lives with joy and happiness. The mechanism used to develop happiness is **"love and warmth"** between children and parents. But love and warmth are abstract. They're invisible. A large number of people haven't realized that having children can bring happiness because they cannot see how happiness will develop from raising children. They can see only visible outcomes, i.e., confusion, exhaustion, and a waste of time and money. Many people avoid having children due to these burdens.

In the past, even though some might not want to have children, as they grow older, they tended to change their minds because, without children, marriage seemed bland and empty. So, many people decided to get married and eventually brought children into their lives. Since then, their lives have changed drastically and generally better.

The degree of happiness depends on how much they love their children. The more they love, the happier they will be. This is because the mechanisms mentioned earlier could function fully. Finally, they started to understand why their parents urged them to have children of their own. But it took them over a decade to realize that.

However, nowadays the situation is no longer the same. There are numerous activities to choose from. A lot of people decided not to have families of their own or not to have children but prefer seeking happiness from activities in the modern world. They find happiness from "pleasure and excitement" through available means. These tools are often concrete and clearly visible, easily attract their attention, and offer pleasure and excitement they want instantly. For example, new models of smartphones, new models of game players, and new forms of entertaining activities. Many decided not to pay attention to "love and warmth" from building a family because they are abstract and invisible. That's why a lot of people think "modern families don't need children." What's the point of making themselves busy by raising children anyway? They seem to know many other ways to enjoy lives. But crucial things they don't realize are **"the importance of family lives"** and **"reasons behind having children."**

Thus, without logical detailed explanations, "having children" — an age-old path of living and a path toward true happiness — may eventually be forgotten, disappear, or become rare. And humans may finally become endangered like pandas because "pleasure and excitement" of the modern world will be more and more arousing and can be found more easily to the point where the importance of building a family will be erased and completely forgotten. In the future, having children may become "something unexpected, strange, or unreasonable."

Due to such ignorance,
many have chosen to live
with "pleasure and excitement"
and use them to drive
their lives without knowing
that the best life drive is
"love and warmth" in the family.

Let's look closely at how things around us work:

- A car will run smoothly and takes more time for its engine to wear out if we use the right engine lubricant.
- Your smartphone will be durable and function properly if you use accessories like a charger and a battery, from the company that made the phone.
- A printer will give a pleasant-looking printout if you use the ink cartridge from the same producer.

This is because genuine accessories, spare parts, and refills were specifically designed for those machines. Thus, they function smoothly and efficiently. And if they come from the same factories, you can be even more confident. Similarly, the body, mind, and love share the same origin which is Nature. They were designed to work in tandem with one another. Driving your life in the direction of family's love and warmth is more in harmony with your body and mind than heading toward pleasure and excitement. As you can see from the previous photos, if those elderly people had chosen to lead their lives in the direction of pleasure and excitement, when they grew older, they would have found that:

- The pleasure and excitement could no longer bring happiness the same way a counterfeit battery cannot last very long.
- Their health might have deteriorated faster or they could have died already. This is because living an adventurous life is hard on your body and there is a risk that you may have an accident. In the same vein, the machine of a car with a wrong kind of lubricant can easily be worn out and damaged.

We can assume that the elderly in the previous picture chose "love and warmth" as his life drive. Therefore, even in his twilight years, he still gains happiness and moral support to fight against problems and obstacles.

A Gift From God or Nature

"Love" is a vital mechanism that Nature uses to guide living things to walk within the path she desires.

To sustain their species continuously. To this end, Nature designs different kinds of love as follows:

- Love of their own lives makes them "fear death." All animals try to stay away from all kinds of harm and dangers so that they can live longer.
- Love and lust lead to matchmaking or marriage, followed by having children.
- Parents' love makes them more concerned about their children's lives than their own. So, the parents try their best to care for and protect their children.

These kinds of love help all kinds of animals including humans survive and sustain their species continuously for hundreds of thousand years. Only a few faced extinctions. All in all, this mechanism has been highly successful.

To make family lives happy. Child-rearing takes more than a decade. During this long period, if the parents are not rewarded with happiness, they may abandon or hurt their children. Thus, Nature makes family lives happy through a variety of mechanisms, e.g., developing a bond and creating the funniest comedians in the world. Even though the parents cannot go out, they still enjoy themselves and find their lives more meaningful than before. Their house is turned into an amusement park. The laughter of family members gets louder and louder when the children have become the greatest comedians of the house. These mechanisms have brought happiness to countless homes throughout the world whether they're rich or poor; live in a big civilized city or a remote town. All parents smile and laugh every day in the comfort of their own homes.

To make the parents want to do good deeds and contribute to society. When a large number of people come to live together for hundreds of thousand years, if they all happen to be selfish and think only about themselves, that society could eventually collapse. Therefore, Nature wants us to do good deeds and support our society to make it a better place. And family love is an important drive for people to contribute to their society.

- Children behave so that they'll be admired by their parents. The fact that they love their parents motivates them to be well-behaved.
- Good behaviors of the parents originate from their desire to set good examples for their beloved children.

- Parents want their children to enjoy a good environment because they love them. They think about the world in the future and try to make it a better place so that their children could have a good quality of life. This is evident in the letter written by Facebook CEO to his daughter the day she was born. "...Like all parents, we want you to grow up in a world better than ours today. ... to join people across the world to advance human potential and promote equality for all children in the next generation. ... We will give 99% of our Facebook shares — currently about $45 billion — during our lives to advance this mission."

Even though this does not happen to everyone and even if we cannot build an ideal world, we can at least counteract the effects of those who are harming the world. The more people focusing on making the world a better place, the fitter it is to live in. And we'll be in a better position to sustain human species and our civilization. This is exactly what Nature wants.

To give the parents moral support in taking care of their families. For the system to be sustainable, it has to be monitored. And people involved need to be rewarded to give them moral support. Nature also takes this principle into account by offering special rewards to those who have been taking good care of their families to encourage them and to sustain the family system as long as possible. If this system collapses, there will be great losses. And the sustainability of human species will be at risk.

In order to bring the "gift" or "reward," Nature has provided certain conditions as follows:

- Nature makes our behaviors work like mirrors. If children have been receiving love from their parents in whatever way, they will love them the same way in return. For example, if parents express their love by hugging and kissing, their children will do the same to show their affection. If parents had rarely spent time with their children, the children would not have time for them either. As the classical physics theory has stated,

"Action = Reaction"

- In our twilight years, we can rarely help ourselves. We'll be like infants who have to depend on others. The difference is that when we were born, Nature gave us caregivers, i.e., our parents. But when we grow old, "Nature makes us seek caregivers by ourselves."

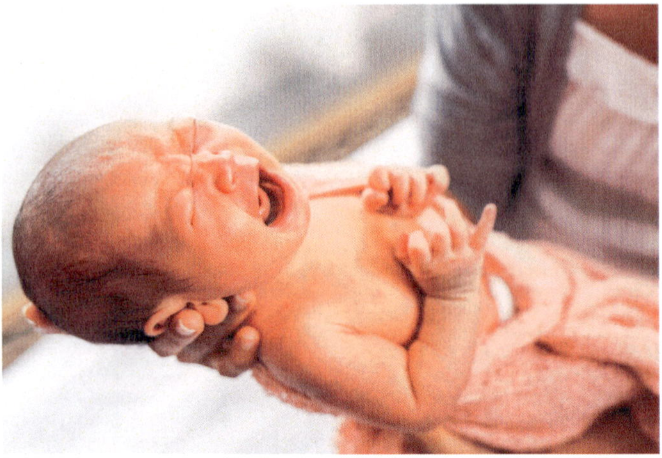

| Newborn babies cannot take care of themselves, so they must depend on their parents for their survival.

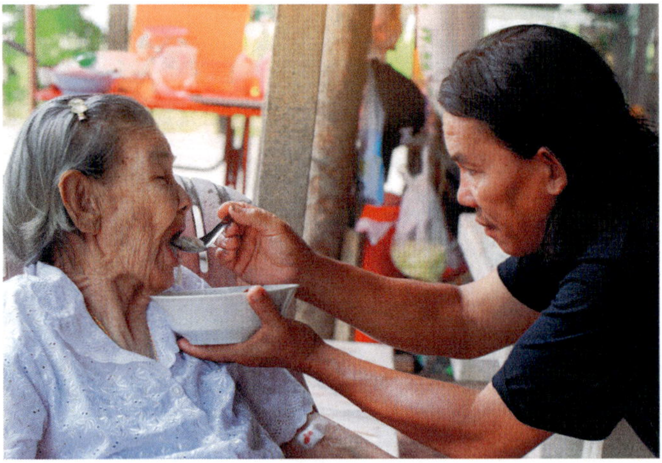

| Elderly people who cannot take care of themselves need help from others.

■ Caregiving is a delicate job. It requires carefulness and attention because infants and some elderly people cannot tell us what they need. The caregivers have to figure out how they feel and what they need.

"Good" caregiving requires caregivers who work with their heart and soul. The power of money or any other kind of power cannot provide good caregiving. Some people may afford to hire others to help take care of their aged parents. However, there must be people (e.g., their own children who truly love them) around to monitor the caregivers to ensure proper caregiving.

These 3 conditions gradually develop "a reward." In the beginning, the parents offer their children love and warmth until they start to "love them back." That is why children feel happy when their parents are happy. As a result, children find ways to make their parents happy such as taking them out for a meal, on a trip, and looking after them as they grow old. This is what we call "gratitude," which emerges naturally. The development of love also creates "a caregiver."

Therefore, a gift that God or Nature intentionally created for parents who had taken care of their family earnestly is "a caregiver" who cares attentively for them. This is not only moral support for the hardworking parents but also functioning as feedback to punish parents who hadn't taken care of their families. Those who abandoned or hurt their children mentally and physically will not receive love in return. Suffice to say, the family system consists of a monitoring system, evaluation, reward and punishment. Thus, this system works efficiently and continues to play an important role in sustaining family institution to this day.

The Main Element of Happiness

Even though family love is one of the abstract matters, it brings countless consequences, e.g., life drive, caregivers (children) who look after their parents earnestly, the greatest comedians in the world, and the sense of wanting to do good deeds. These are good things in our lives. Furthermore, family love is an important and the oldest source of happiness for humans. This is because early on humans did not have any other sources of happiness. Although it was the only source, it gave them warmth and entertainment. They laughed every day and several times a day and saw the world as a delightful place to be. Even when they were facing fatal crises, family love encouraged them to get through those tough times. This fact of life has been going on for hundreds of thousand years along with human species. The same holds true today, which can be observed in remote areas far away from civilization. Despite the lack of electricity and water supply; entertainment places; Internet to follow the news or download games, they still live a happy life due to love and warmth from their families.

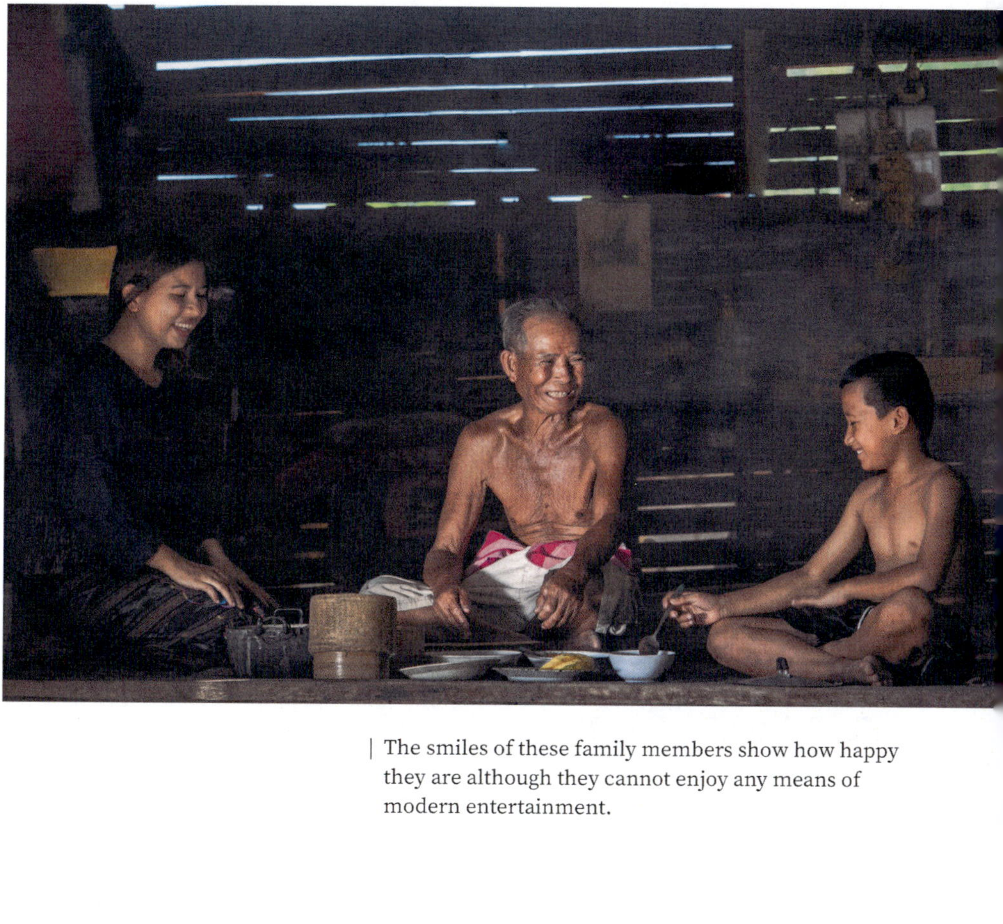

The smiles of these family members show how happy they are although they cannot enjoy any means of modern entertainment.

Happiness can happen to everyone whether the person is rich or poor; lives in a big city or a remote area. If you have a loving home, you can enjoy a happy life. This does not only happen with humans, but most animals also enjoy this kind of happiness as can be seen in the pictures below:

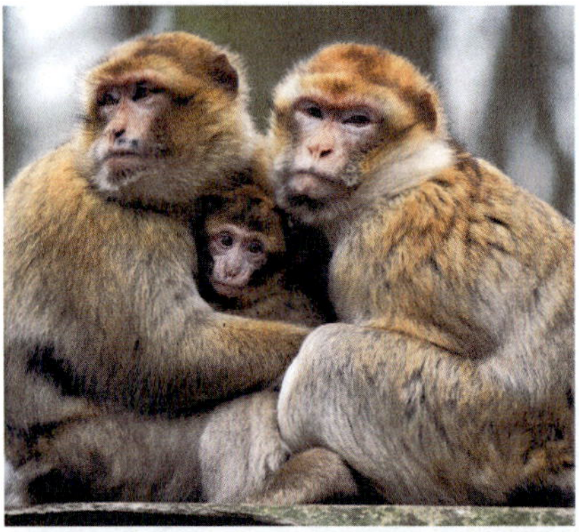

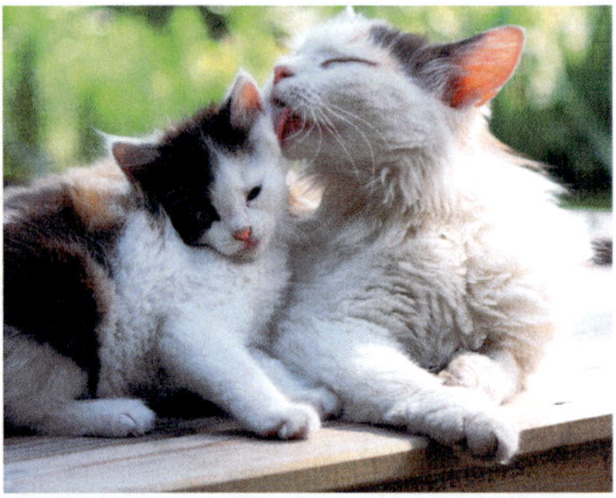

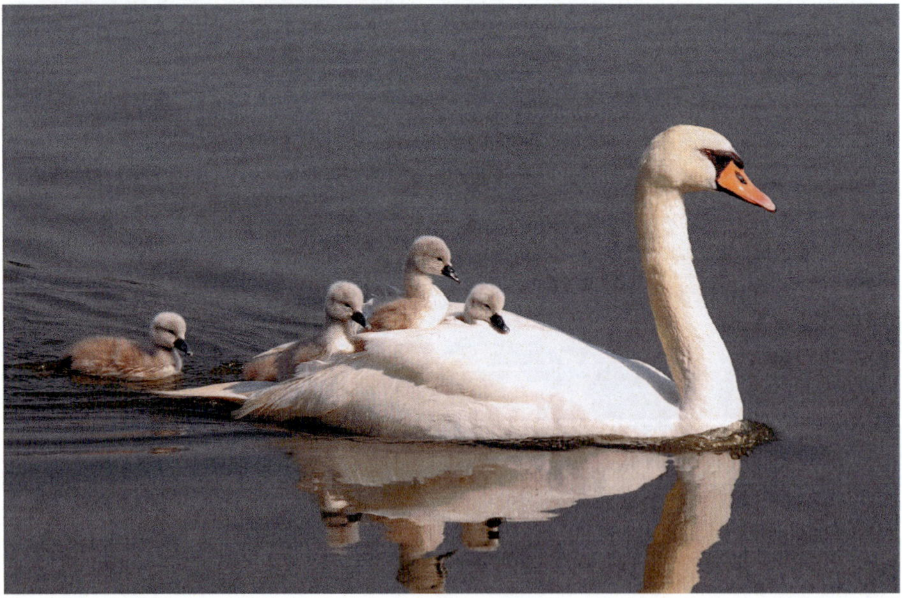

Family warmth is an important mechanism to achieve happiness in life although other factors may be lacking. As time has passed by and the world has become more and more civilized. Everything in our environment has been developed, modified, and modernized. Our lives have been adjusted to be more comfortable and luxurious. Therefore, happiness in a family also looks different as can be seen in the pictures below:

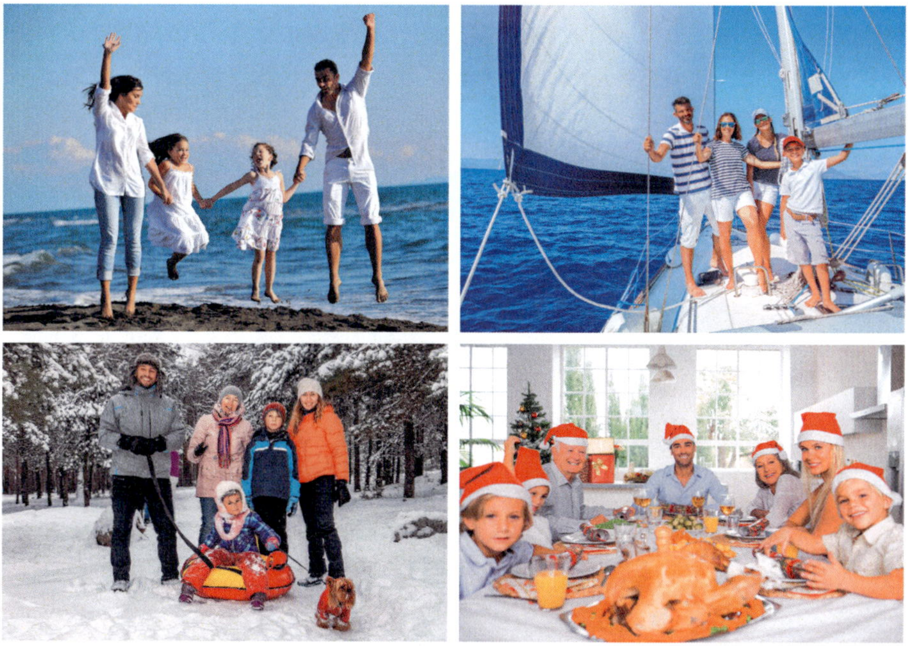

| Modern family lives

Sometimes our environment has been modified so much that the original elements or "love and warmth" that used to bring true happiness to families become invisible. Some examples of what have been over-modified are as follows:

- Cruising in a luxurious yacht or using an extremely expensive car just to look chic.
- Obsession with unnecessary things, e.g., games and gambling.
- Leading a luxurious lifestyle such as collecting jewelry and owning extremely expensive houses.

No matter how much these things are modified, they simply just add colors to lives. They don't change the original mechanism of happiness-building and can never replace "love and warmth in the family" which remain the important elements for developing happiness in humans and animals. These modifications are like adding colors to your dish by a chef to make the food looks better and more appetizing like a dish of fried rice in the pictures below:

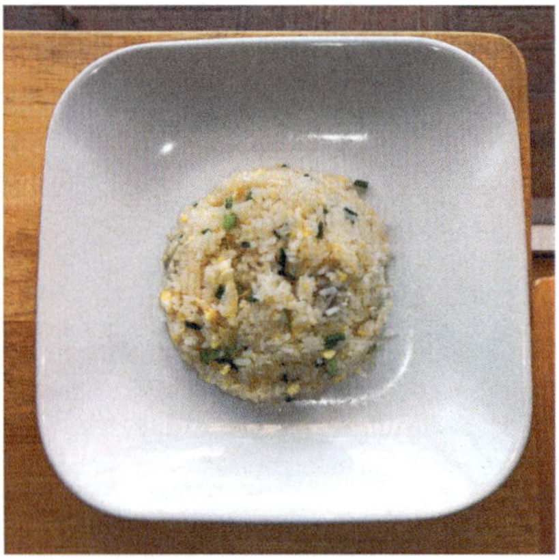

| A dish of fried rice before adding garnishes

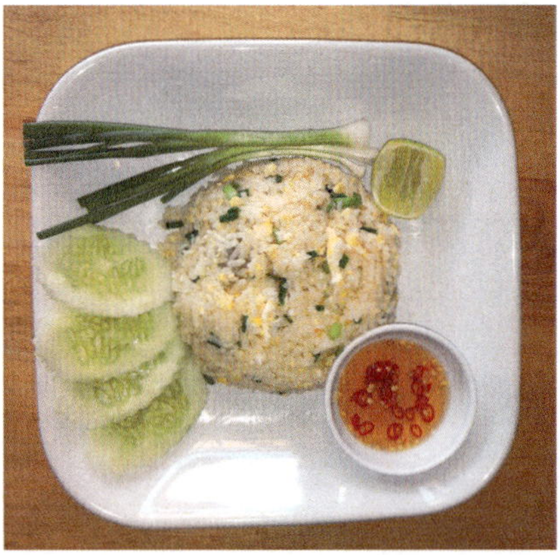

| A dish of fried rice after adding garnishes

No matter how we decorate the dish, the main element is still "fried rice." This fact is very important because it's what we depend on when choosing our path of living. When we grow up, at some point we will have to decide whether we want to stay single or get married.

The ability to distinguish between the main elements and the garnishes will lead us to choose the best paths for our lives.

People who know nothing about "garnishes" usually think their property like big houses, beautiful cars, and amusing computer games brings happiness to lives. This is because they are influenced by all kinds of media around them portraying that these things are the sources of happiness. Although it's not necessarily inaccurate, it's only partly true. Money, houses, cars, and computer games are only garnishes. They just make lives more colorful and will function quite well as long as there are the main elements. On the contrary, if there are only these garnishes, they cannot do much contributing to a person's happiness, as you can see in the picture below:

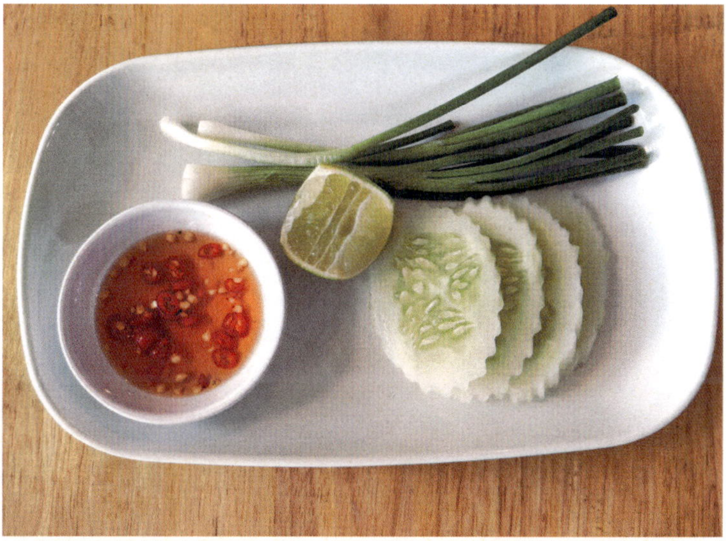

| Garnishes without the main element

The function of garnishes is merely to decorate the dish. Without the main element, they are rather powerless. Therefore, people with money, expensive houses, and luxurious cars (garnishes) who do not have warm and loving families cannot discover complete happiness. Because they are still missing the more important elements for a happy life. The following pictures will illustrate this point more clearly:

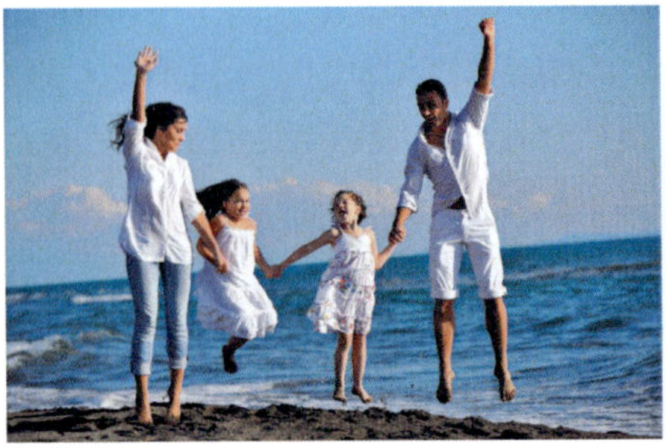

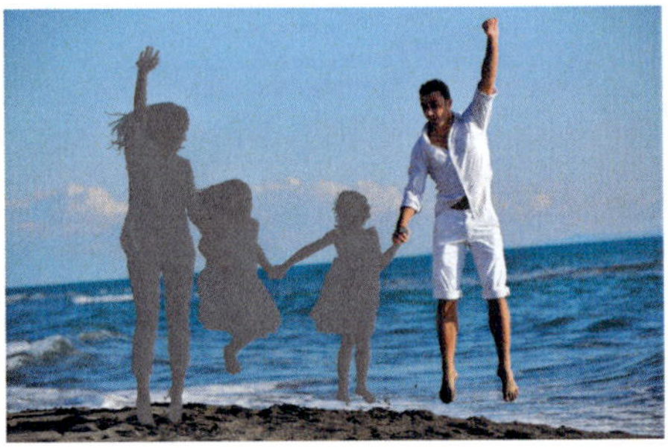

The man in the picture on the left is happy because he's spending time with his family. But if everyone else is missing and he is the only one left, his happiness will definitely decrease. Even though he was still on the same beach, he probably wouldn't jump up with joy like that. In addition, he might not even walk out of his hotel room to stroll on the beach because walking alone is not fun. In this case, only the garnish or the beach cannot bring him so much happiness.

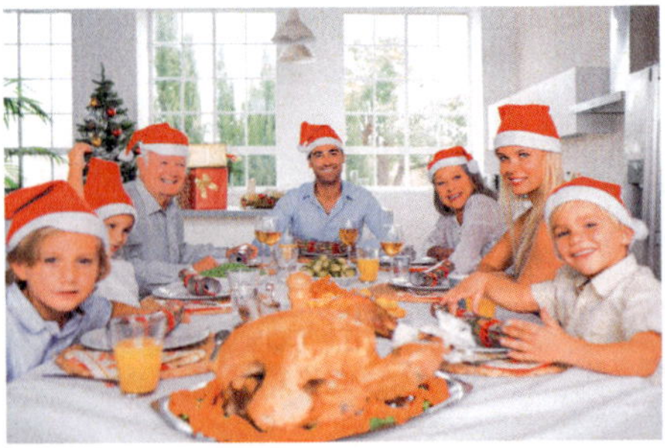

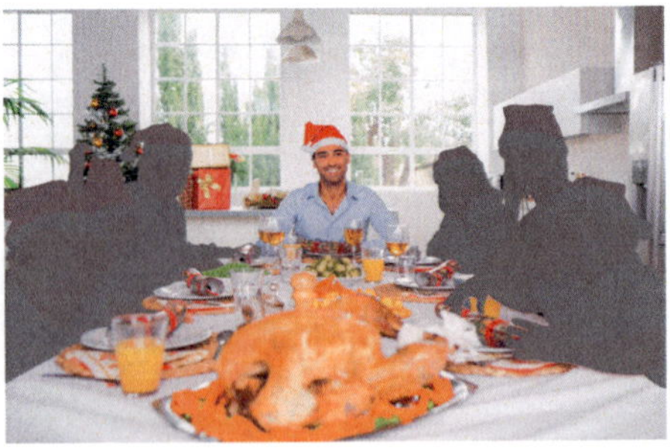

Everyone is enjoying a delicious meal in a warm environment. But if everyone else was missing, the man at the end of the table wouldn't be as cheerful. Although the same set of meal was still there, his smile would possibly disappear. And it's quite intriguing that the turkey on the right wouldn't be as delicious as the one on the left although it is the same turkey.

Without the main element or a warm family, the garnishes cannot function at their full potential. Garnishes that make lives more colorful, e.g., money, houses, cars, food, and tourist attractions will bring much more joy when the main element is already there. To sum up, a warm family brings complete happiness to life because people can enjoy both the main element and its garnishes.

Since family love brings along several consequences. Choosing not to have kids eliminates these "consequences," in other words, not having the funniest comedian in the world and the caregiver. Without a family, you're likely to lead a lonely life because there will be no joker to bring laughter. And upon entering your twilight years, there will be no caregivers who will play the most meaningful role in your life.

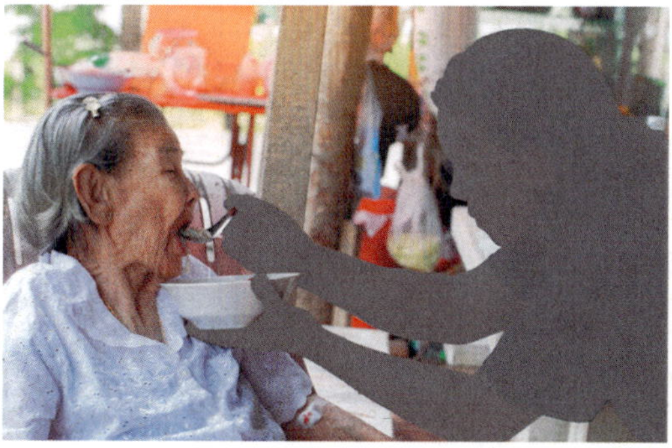

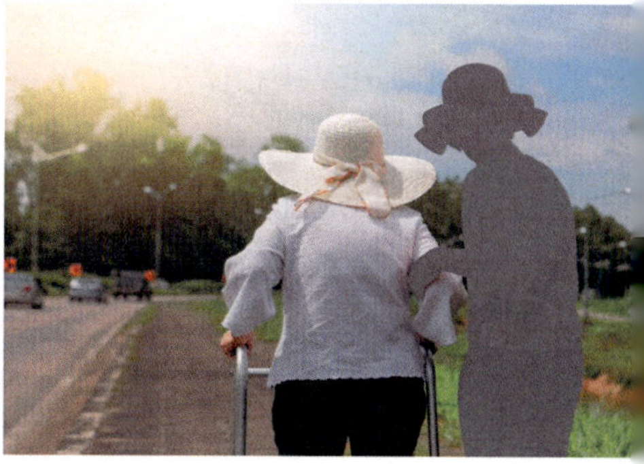

One Way or Another, We Struggle for Happiness

In this chapter, I will discuss what may be called the "disadvantages" of building a family rather than its advantages.

Despite its importance and many advantages, having a loving family involves a process that is rather abstract and goes on quietly, there seems to be nothing special. That's why many people do not realize the advantages of it. Due to this kind of ignorance, what goes on in each family seems hidden. Actually, it's not. It's just that the majority of people are not aware of reasons to have a family and do not realize that having children can bring happiness. And now that we've entered the age of high-speed Internet, people are preoccupied with their smartphones. Even when they're having a meal together, they tend to pay attention to their phones instead of each other. Meanwhile, "having children" turns out to be more and more far-fetched to the point where some people say "a modern family doesn't need children."

Therefore, it is vital that this book shines a spotlight on family lives, a system built and designed particularly for mankind, so the readers can see how valuable it is.

The fact that family happiness is intangible is one of the drawbacks. As it turns out, "an important matter" has become "something trivial" for most people. Furthermore, building a warm and loving family is rather difficult because it requires several factors. This kind of difficulty also counts as a disadvantage.

The first drawback, ignorance, has led a large number of people to decide not to get married. Some enter into a marriage but avoid having children. The second drawback is the difficulty of building a truly warm and loving family. That is, many people look forward to building a family, but they fail to do so and become disappointed and upset because:

- They cannot find a boy/girlfriend.
- Those with boy/girlfriend eventually terminate their relationship, causing some people to commit suicide.
- Some couples stayed married for years without having children although they've resorted to countless in vitro fertilization.

Our lives are complex and related to a large number of factors. People who are successful and fulfilled in all aspects of their lives don't exist. Everyone has to face disappointments one way or another. When disappointments (e.g., getting dumped; being heartbroken; facing unemployment; falling gravely ill) emerge, we have to deal with them so that they won't ruin our entire lives. We have to continue leading our lives even though we're confronted with disappointment. And importantly, we have to lead happy lives. Some methods have been proven to successfully deal with disappointments and bring happiness, for example:

- Be optimistic, focusing on what we have, not what we're lacking.
- Don't obsess over what we cannot change.

Building a family and having children are good things. However, if you cannot have them, you should try to forget about them. And this book may no longer be interesting to you because it's suitable for those who are choosing whether to get married and have children or not. Unless you want to learn about Nature's secrets of building a family, you can put this book down.

Not only does this book offer knowledge about choosing a path of living but it's also suitable for those who are taking care of their children. During this period, they'll have to face a number of unexpected and unexplainable situations. For example, why is raising children so tiring and time-consuming? Or why are children so mischievous? These unanswered questions might stay in their subconscious, which may eventually put them in a bad mood. This book will explain these situations and help the readers understand them. Then this understanding will help family members lead their lives happily together.

Therefore, this book is just like a user's manual in a package of a new electric appliance. The manual is very important since it explains to you in detail the proper use and how to keep the appliance in a good condition for a long time. This book is a manual for those with families. Its content aims at offering a better understanding of family lives and helping you lead a happy family. So it is essential that people with families read this book thoroughly.

How Does Nature Motivate Us to Have Children?

In the first section,
you've learned about
the mechanisms
Nature plans to make
"having children"
a favorable path of living.
Since everyone starts
as a single person,
Nature needs to build
additional mechanisms
to encourage humans
to choose not to stay "single"
and enter the path that
will lead them to "bringing
children into the world."
So, in the next pages,
I will discuss these
mechanisms in detail.

The 3 Paths of Living
and Other Interesting Points

In this book, lifestyles are
divided into 3 forms:
1. Living with parents (or staying single)
2. Getting married without children, and
3. Getting married with children

Path 1: Living With Parents

If you look at the works of Nature carefully, you will see that each is complex and involves a number of mechanisms. Even scientists with expertise in each area cannot understand half of the mechanisms working behind the scenes, as shown in the following examples:

- How our organs work, e.g., the brain, kidney, and immune system.
- Disasters such as an earthquake and a volcanic eruption. (A simple question like "when will these things happen and end?" cannot yet be answered.)
- Almost everything about our solar system.

Similarly, "having children" is complicated and there are many things involved that we don't know about. However, if things go wrong, it means the extinction of the human species. That's why Nature had to meticulously design this path of life by rigorously plan related mechanisms to ensure that "having children" will continue endlessly.

This job is not something that can be achieved easily. "Having children" involves troubles and exhaustion. Thus, a large number of people don't choose this path of living. Motivating humans to have children must be done ingeniously. Furthermore, during a particular period, they're enjoying the comfort of their safe and warm homes where their parents are taking good care of them. This makes it twice harder to convince them to shift to a new path of "having their own children" because they have to abandon the comfort and start a new life full of troubles and exhaustion.

But Nature solves this problem with ease by offering a second path that is attractive, colorful, and exciting. It is the path enriched by "young love," the kind of love designed particularly for this job. People in love are always delighted and joyful. They see the world as such a wonderful place to live. Young love also creates happiness they've never experienced before. They will feel as if they were the only two people on earth. And they see their "young love" as the most precious thing.

Not only does young love bring happiness, but it also affects other parts of their lives. When a couple has fallen in love, living with their parents starts to feel uncomfortable, uninteresting, dull and boring. Under the watchful eyes of their parents, they think they don't have freedom and independence. So, they no longer want to have this kind of lifestyle. They want a new kind that includes "young love" and will try every way they can to make this happen. Even though they may be interfered with, discouraged, or interrupted by their friends and relatives, they're still determined to achieve this goal. A person in love can be as stubborn as a mule.

This means that Nature can eventually change our path of living, shifting from living with parents to starting our own family "with children." Because the road decorated with "young love" is right next to the path that leads to "having children." When young people entered this path of love, it means they're leaning toward the idea of "having children."

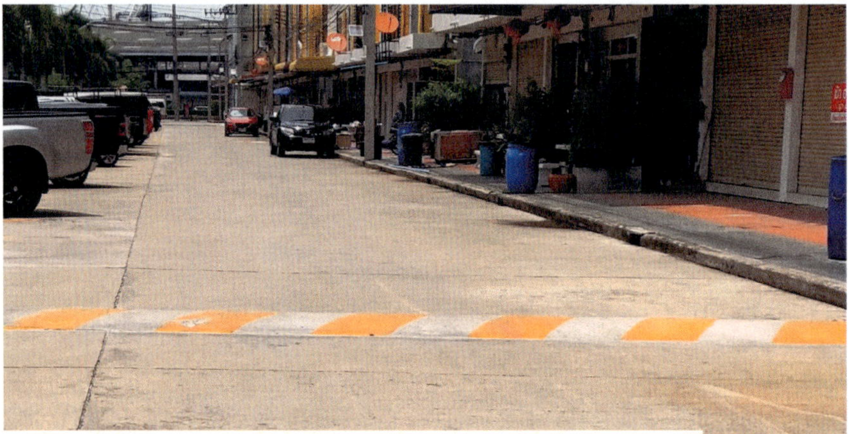

A speed bump

If you look carefully, you'll see that Nature changes our course of living by decorating the new path to look so attractive it's hard to resist. On the other hand, she places speed bumps, i.e., frustration and boredom on the previous path to form the feeling that it is no longer fit to walk on. This way, Nature can control our destiny at will. In fact, the transition designed by Nature is smooth and powerful because it matches the desire in our hearts.

Nature and Mechanisms Behind the Scenes

There are many movie scenes, whether it's an action scene, a scene where an actor is chased by a dinosaur, a war scene, or a love scene. All these scenes look realistic and make us feel like we were a part of those events, as shown in the picture below:

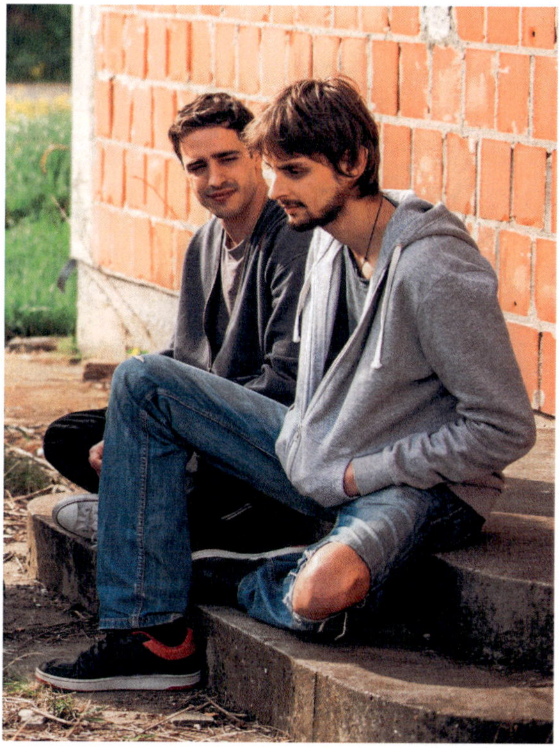

To complete each scene in a movie requires several teams of experts, for example, actors, the director and his crew, make-up artists, costume crew, and those who take care of miscellaneous tasks like moving a camera; holding a microphone; carrying a reflector. These are people you don't see in the movie.

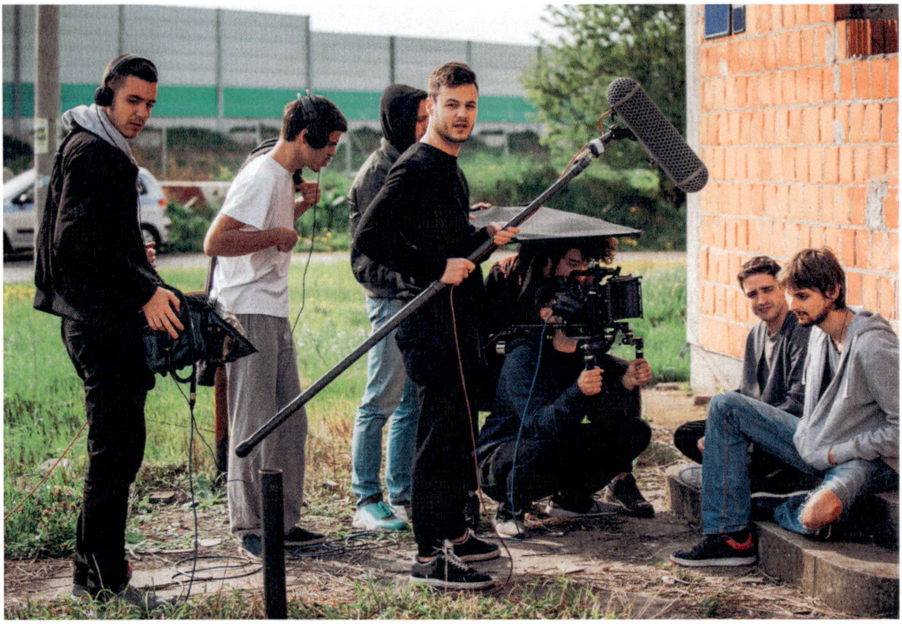

What you see in each scene is an outcome of these efficient teams of people who have to work harmoniously to achieve it. And this will happen only when there is a wonderful plan. Likewise, creating "young love," a small abstract matter, is not easy. For this "young love" to be activated, there must be several changes:

- The body must grow rapidly and start to possess the characteristics of an adult.
- The sexual organs and different kinds of hormones start to change rapidly.

- Moods, thoughts, and feelings change tremendously as if he/she was another person. For example, when the person was a child, he always stayed with his parents and often asked to accompany them wherever they went. But upon turning into a teenager, he would prefer to be alone or with his friends. It could be said that at that point he loves his friends more than his parents.

These changes turn a lovely small child into a totally different teenager. The person seems to change completely. This is similar to turning a tadpole into a frog because these two phenomena create new incredible things. Finally, these changes bring about "young love."

Both turning a tadpole into a frog and creating "young love" take several steps, requiring great planning on the creator's part. The creator or Nature must have prepared well in advance by building "commands" within humans' genes since they were born. And when the time is right, the "commands" will start to work for these changes to take place.

Although "young love" develops in such a meticulous and complicated way, "young love" itself cannot change our lives to the point Nature wants. Similarly, a movie cannot be complete with only one scene. Therefore, Nature needs to create other scenes to lead our lives to the climax or Nature's goal. That is, "bring children into the world." I will discuss these other scenes including things going on behind the scenes in detail in the next section.

Path 2: Young Love and Its Problems

When young people have entered the 2nd path, what Nature has to do is guide them toward the 3rd path. That is "a family with children." To this end, Nature resorts to the same technique – "decorating the path to look so beautiful to attract these young people. Meanwhile, speed bumps are placed in the previous path to make them feel that it is no longer pleasant to walk on." What Nature brings to decorate the 3rd path is still "love." But it's different from the kind of love used to decorate the 2nd path and even more superior to "young love." No one will be willing to shift to this new route unless they find something more satisfactory.

As you may notice, although "young love" is tempting and fascinating, it may lead to problems more often than to happiness:

- Your lover may not love only one person. He/she may be seeing someone else at the same time. In fact, your lover may even have 3 - 4 lovers at the same time. (two-timing)
- Some couples had lived together for several years, but when one of them found someone else better-looking or richer, he/she just left shamelessly as if nothing happened. (unfaithfulness)
- Some people are heartbroken because they are not loved in return. Love may turn into rage, causing them to attack or even kill the other person. (violence)
- Some couples may live together for benefits, not because of love. For example, hoping for money, fame, or business interests. (valuing money over love)
- Some quarrel with or even attack each other regularly. They don't even dare to look at each other's faces because doing so may cause the other to think that they want to fight. Some might be beaten daily. (living miserable and fearful lives)
- Although a couple had lived together for a decade, when one suffered a misfortune, e.g., falling ill or losing a job and regular income, the person who used to say "we will grow old together" just left. (being left when faced with misfortune)

So, a large number of people are afraid of "love." Many developed mental illness or paranoia. They no longer trust anyone throughout their lives. Some went bankrupt because they were cheated. Some committed suicide.

This is because there are some "flaws" hidden in their relationship that cause recurring problems. These "flaws" are nothing else but "dark sides" in our hearts that are usually greed, selfishness, cruelty, and malice. The problems caused by these "flaws" or "dark sides" will get more and more severe as shown in the following examples:

- Initially, a person may get beaten slightly. But the longer they stay together, the stronger the beating to the point of bleeding or getting seriously injured.
- In the beginning, a boy/girlfriend may borrow just a small amount of money. But the longer they remain a couple, the more money is borrowed and never returned. Finally, the money reserved for an emergency is gone.

Not only do the problems get more serious but "dark sides" also keep emerging. Eventually, the characteristics and behaviors of that person change as if he/she were a different person, from someone lovely and gentle to a person who is quick-tempered, cruel, and selfish. At that point, no one can see the love once resided in his/her heart.

Because love and darkness within a person share the same natural foundation. Both are feelings in a person's heart. Therefore, when one emotion is stronger, the other naturally fades. Similarly, the love in someone's heart gets weaker and is overcome by that person's dark sides until love disappears completely.

Diluting something valuable by adding something worthless to it is the same as adulteration of goods, e.g., adulterated gasoline; shampoos; fertilizer. Love that has been adulterated is often recognized as faded love, untrue love, phony love, or impure love.

Only true love or pure love brings happiness to lives, yet it's hard to avoid problems of adulteration. Since seeking true or pure love is difficult, love lives of young people often bring unfavorable outcomes. Couples with deeply adulterated love usually end up in divorce. One with less adulteration can live together, but with difficulty. Their love is often on and off. Sometimes they're sweet with each other, the other times they fight. Those who can find true or pure love will have a smooth and peaceful relationship. However, this rarely happens. That's why divorce and violence in families occur regularly around the world.

Nevertheless, true or pure love is the most desirable thing among young people. They struggle to find it even though in the end all they've found is untrue love with all kinds of problems. They are not discouraged, give up, or change their minds and hope that one true love will come to them and they'll live happily ever after.

Path 3: Turning Family Lives Into a Path of Happiness

As I've explained, young couples rarely survive on the 2nd path (family lives without children). Walking on the 3rd path (getting married and having children) is even harder and the chance to be successful is much less. But Nature wants them to enter this 3rd path. Therefore, she must help them get through possible obstacles.

On this new path, the married couples are accompanied by their children. It means they have more responsibilities, especially families with several children like 3 - 5 children. In the past, some families had as many as 10 children. There are so many more long-lasting responsibilities. It takes more than a decade for each kid to grow up. Walking on the 3rd path is, therefore, many times more laborious than the 2nd path.

This long-lasting exhaustion negatively affects their journey. Even married couples without children (those on the 2nd path) who do not have to take care of anyone else but themselves can rarely succeed in their relationship. If they also have to be responsible for their children, it's hard to imagine how they can manage to survive this new path.

However, the 3rd path is Nature's ultimate goal. Because if no one enters this route, the human race will face extinction. Therefore, Nature lends a hand to make sure they'll survive this new path by planning solutions for different problems that will appear along the way.

- Having to travel a long journey: The fact that they have to be on this path for more than a decade might make them get so bored or discouraged that they decide to give up. Ending the journey will definitely have negative effects on sustaining the species. So, Nature offers "the funniest comedian in the world," as explained earlier, to accompany them. This comedian will bring laughter along the journey. Although this journey is long and exhausting, it's amusing and joyful. As a result, time flies quickly and we often hear these parents say "Look at them. The next thing I know, my children have become teenagers."
- Obstacles along the 3rd path: These obstacles, e.g., troubles, exhaustion, and discouragement are related to child-rearing. Thus, Nature assists them by providing shields or armors to protect them.

Nature provides these gifts, i.e., laughter and shields or armors through a mechanism called "love." She designs a new kind of love for these parents – love between parents and children – to be pure and genuine. This is because Nature realizes what will happen when this kind of love exists in their lives.

And since the love between parents and children is "genuine" and "pure," it's not contaminated by "dark sides" such as greed, selfishness, cruelty, and malice. So, it can bring endless joy that will not be interfered with or interrupted like "young love" on the 2nd path. Moreover, they don't have to face negative consequences that accompany the dark sides, e.g., lying, two-timing, abandoning, and violence. Therefore, their love develops gradually and continuously until it eventually fills their hearts. The following pictures show parents with children (members of the 3rd path) who are facing problems or obstacles:

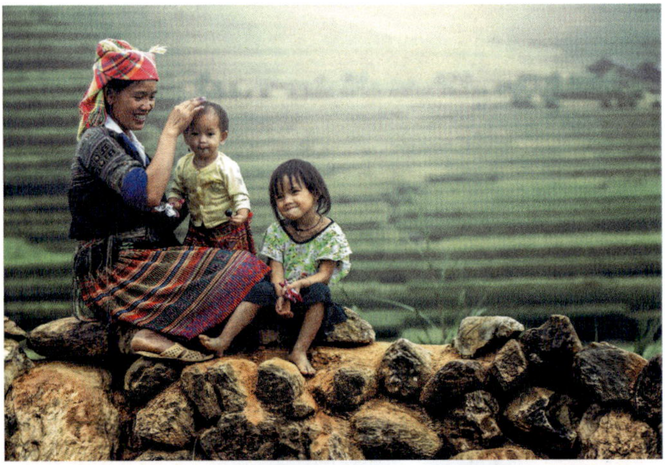

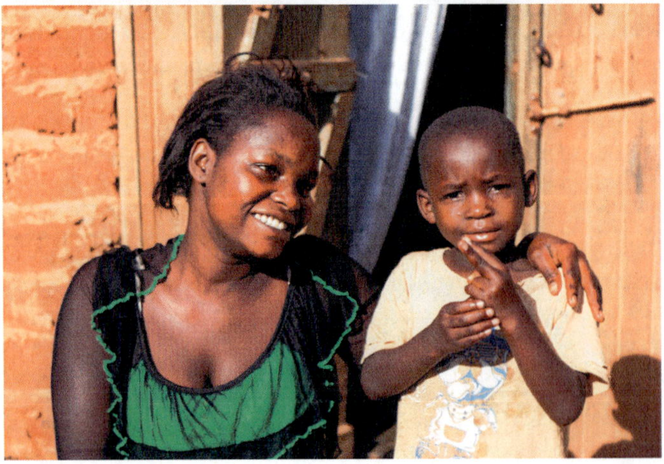

Those trapped in poverty or living in remote areas away from civilization lack food, medicine, electricity, and water supply.

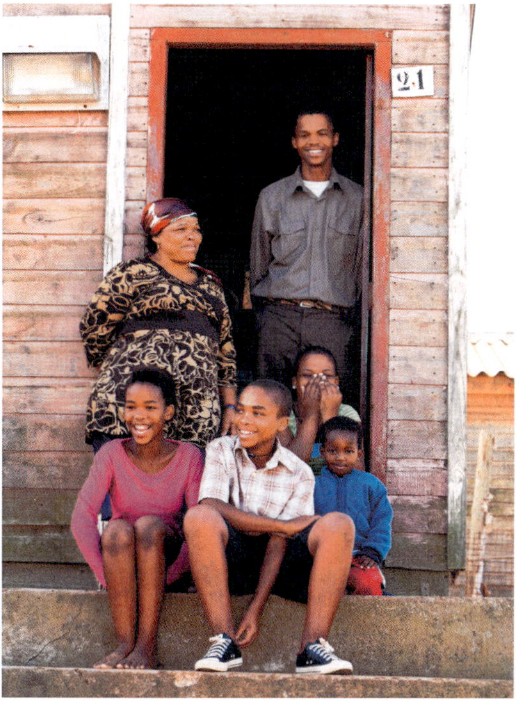

A family with several children is rather crowded. They have to share everything such as food, chairs, beds, and especially bathrooms, (competing to use a bathroom or using it at the same time). This may lead to frustration and a lack of privacy.

Even though "having children" brings all kinds of headaches, they can still lead happy lives as you can see the smiles on their faces:

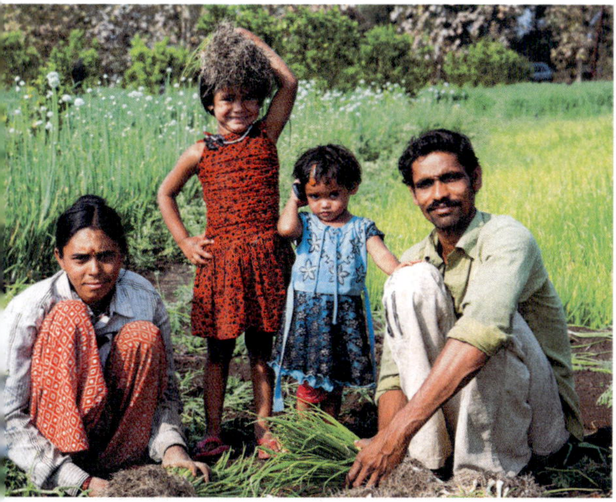

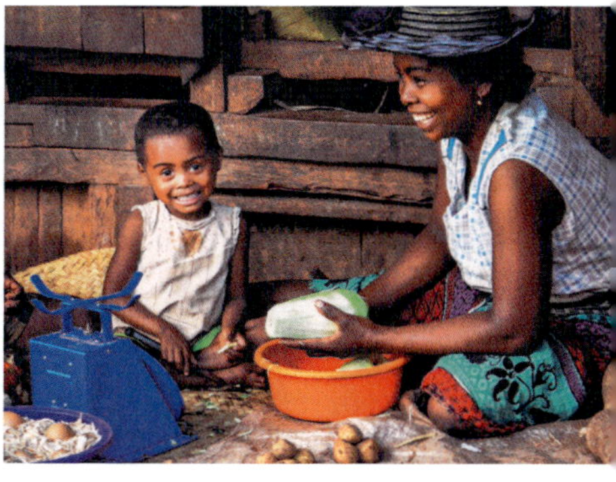

Working to financially support themselves and their families (including their children) can lead to stress, fatigue, and discouragement.

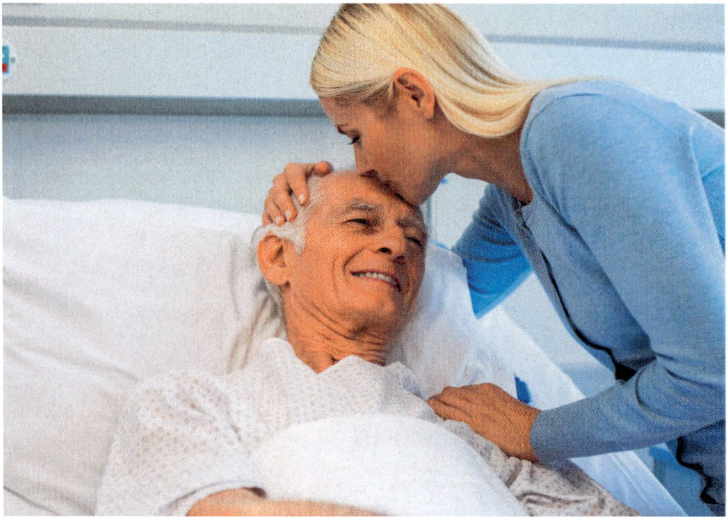

Growing old and getting sick may cause worries and fear.

It's rather "unusual" to be happy while facing all kinds of problems. Naturally, we suffer when confronting unfavorable circumstances. The more problems we have to deal with, the more we suffer. Thus, it's hard to believe families with children (those walking on the 3rd path) will enjoy their lives because they have to face far more unfavorable situations, e.g., troubles, exhaustion, discouragement, stress, fear, and worries.

However, this 3rd path is the only path that will help humans sustain their species. Nature has to keep them happy while walking on this road of lives by ensuring that those unsatisfactory circumstances will not interrupt their journey. And although these situations occur quite often, Nature can deal with each of them all at once by using an approach that seems quite simple but has a deep aspect hidden inside. On the surface, this approach seems weird, incredible, and impossible, the kind of feelings that emerge when you hear an answer for a trick question or as the proverb has it, "Some people cannot see the wood for the trees." But when reflecting deeply upon this approach, one will see that it's a shrewd and great move because time has proved that this approach has been keeping those on the 3rd path happy for hundreds of thousand years or since the dawn of human race.

This approach is based on the fact that unfavorable things on the 3rd path (whether it's trouble, exhaustion, discouragement, frustration, stress, fear, or worries) are all feelings. These reside in humans' hearts and affect their hearts. Therefore, Nature manages to "shut the gate to the heart" by filling it with love so unfavorable things cannot enter. They can affect them only on the surface.

At this moment, you probably understand why Nature has designed the love between parents and their children to be genuine and pure. Nature wants their love to continue endlessly without being interrupted or being on and off like "young love" on the 2nd path. When time passes by, this kind of love will fill their hearts completely.

Now that you've learned about these facts, please return to the previous pages to look at those family pictures again. This time, you'll see things that you've never seen before. Things that are "abstract" like a number of unfavorable things along these people's path of living and the love residing in their hearts. These are hard to prove and invisible. Yet, there is important evidence confirming that these things exist. That is the "happy smiles" on their faces.

And when we combine what I've described with the idea that "heaven is wherever you find happiness," we can say that true or genuine love, which God or Nature has intentionally created, will make the trouble-filled path more pleasant and enjoyable to walk on.

What Is Pure Love?

Origin and Background

Case Study

Revealing the Truth
Behind the Pure Love of Children

When we talk about "pure love," people in general often think about "a mother's love." This is because a mother's love is full of giving and sacrifice. A mother can do anything for her child without thinking about how much sweat she has to put into it. As long as her child is happy, she will be glad to do it. A mother's act of giving is great and pure. She has begun giving even before the child was born. Her flesh and blood formed the child's body and different organs. After giving birth, she had to take care of her child until they grew up into a good person of the society. Children become who they are because of their mothers. So, a mother's love is great and pure. And because many of us have experienced this kind of love; we understand it completely and think of it when it comes to pure love.

But there is another kind of "true love" or "pure love." Although this kind of love is not as great as "a mother's love" but it is crucial to our lives. Pure love brings happiness to anyone it touches. People who are involved with true love will not have to suffer terrible things such as lies, deceptions, two-timing, abandonment, and assaults. They can enjoy true love without worries. Here I'm talking about "love from children to their parents." People rarely know that this kind of love is also genuine and pure, so this book must explain it in detail to help the readers understand it clearly.

Origin and Background

In a medical school, before students can graduate, they have to be trained in a score of departments or wards and the large and very important one is the children's ward. I can still remember the time when I studied in this ward quite clearly. The professors were experts in the field, so they could teach very fluently, deeply, and enjoyably. The department of pediatrics is divided into different fields, e.g., pediatric infectious diseases, child development, and childhood brain disorders. One thing that all students noticed was that our professors were unusually kind. Oftentimes, while teaching, they would be smiling or even laughing. It was so different from some other departments where professors were very strict. We concluded that this was because they spent most of their time with children. They had to play with their patients to get those children in a good mood so the patients wouldn't give them a hard time during the treatment.

The most important point that our professors emphasized was that "children are not little adults" or "children are not a miniature version of adults." This means that the bodily functions of children and adults are quite different. Some work in the same way; others are completely different. Thus, children's responses to the stimulants may be quite different from adults'. Giving medical treatment requires an understanding of their bodily functions. One must not assume that "because adults' bodies function this way, so do the children's." Some of the differences are as follows:

- Certain medicines cause drowsiness in adults. But if children take them, they could be restless and hyperactive.
- Some diseases found among adults will not appear in children. And some of the children's diseases are not found in adults.
- Some medicines that can be used in adults must not be administered to children due to their side effects, e.g., turning their teeth yellow for the rest of their lives or causing them to be short (because the medicine stops their bone growth).

Children's bodies are going through changes in the process of development. This process takes more than 10 years to complete. While these changes are taking place, their bodies do not function in the same way as adults and also respond to stimulants differently. They'll become teenagers when they're around 15 years old and their bodies will start to function like adults'.

Child development involves the process that is not only physical but psychological. Therefore, when a child's psychological development is not yet complete, his/her emotion and feelings will not be the same as an adult's. This is also true in the case of love. Children's love is not the same as those of adults because emotions and feelings that come with their love are different. This is why children's love is **"true"** or **"pure."** The following case would illustrate my point:

Case Study

Whenever I have a chance, I'll read the magazine called "Khu Sang Khu Som" (Perfect Partners) because there are always life lessons that I can learn from. One day I came across the following article that helped me understand the "pure love" of children more clearly.

This article was released in the 37th year of the magazine (issue 946). The following content was quoted verbatim:

A tragic event occurred recently. While a man was cleaning his new car, his 6-year-old boy wanted to help by picking up a piece of rock and rubbed the hood with it.

Out of rage, the man held his son's hand tightly with one hand and used the other to hit the boy's hand with all his strength without being aware that he was holding a wrench. Even though his son was screaming in pain, he didn't stop.

At the hospital, all the boy's beaten fingers had to be removed because they were too severely injured to treat. When he woke up and realized that his fingers were cut off. He looked at his father with fear in his eyes before softly asking him,

'Dad, will my fingers grow back?'

The father was deeply heart-broken. He was speechless, avoided his son's eye contact and rushed out of the room. Then, he stood aimlessly beside his car and released his temper by kicking it several times before collapsing and sitting on the ground right next to the car. When he managed to control his temper eventually, he looked around and saw the boy's handwriting which caused the boy to be punished. It was unclear but readable:

I love you, dad.

The next day, the father committed suicide.

(I would like to thank Mr.Damrong Phuttan, the magazine's editor-in-chief, for allowing me to use this article.)

We can learn about a number of things from this case. But I'll discuss it in the next section so that the content of this part will not be too lengthy.

Revealing the Truth Behind Pure Love of Children

The case study above offers some valuable lessons as follows:

Pure love of children: How it is formed and some considerations about this kind of love

You can see that even though the child was attacked so violently, he didn't respond or fight back in any way. In this type of situation, all children do is "cry loudly in pain." The only thing that will protect them is mercy from adults. What they can do is begging for their parents' sympathy until the parents stop hurting them. And while crying, they often shout something like "I'm scared" and "Please stop beating me. I won't do it again." No matter how painful it is, children will stand still and accept the punishment without fighting back.

If a violent attack (until fingers' bones were broken like in the case study) occurs with an adult, naturally the person wouldn't allow the attacker to beat him/her up without fighting back. That person would respond or fight back in an equally violent way.

Children don't respond because they don't possess malice or cruelty (or one of the dark sides) in their hearts. Usually what they have are:

- Fear. Nature creates fear to make children particularly careful so they could avoid dangers. In this case study, even though the boy was attacked so badly his fingers had to be surgically removed, all he did was showing his "fear." As shown in the narrative that "He looked at his father with fear in his eyes."
- Curiosity. Children have to learn about a number of things so Nature gives them curiosity. They're always curious and asking questions endlessly. From the case study, when he realized that his fingers were gone, instead of getting angry, he asked his father, "Dad, will my fingers grow back?"

Since children don't possess darkness inside their hearts, i.e., greed, selfishness, cruelty, and malice. With gentleness and friendliness, they're not a threat to people around them. Similarly, the kind of love they express is pure and genuine so it doesn't cause problems the way "young love" does. In general, each child has the same mindset (without dark sides), they express themselves so similarly we can conclude that these are identities of children.

- They love only their parents. They don't just change their mind and love other kids' parents or anyone else more than their own. They're sincere. They're never two-timing.

- They don't deceive their parents. Sometimes they may lie about trivial things to avoid punishment or to get new toys. But they never think about deceiving or hurting their parents.
- They don't value money over love. For children, their priority is always love. The second place is likely to be "toys" or "food." So, it's not surprising to see "I love you, Dad." on the car hood. This is because their hearts are full of "love."

Sincerity, gentleness, and purity make their love "true" and "pure," which will not cause negative effects, e.g., lies, deceptions, two-timing, and abandonment. This kind of love continues without being interrupted or going on and off like young love on the 2nd path. Therefore, their love increases continuously until their parents' hearts are full of love as well.

Pure love of children and the need to change

The outside world is full of dangers and cruelty. Naturally, the weak fall victim to the strong like the antelope that is about to be the cheetah's meal in the picture below:

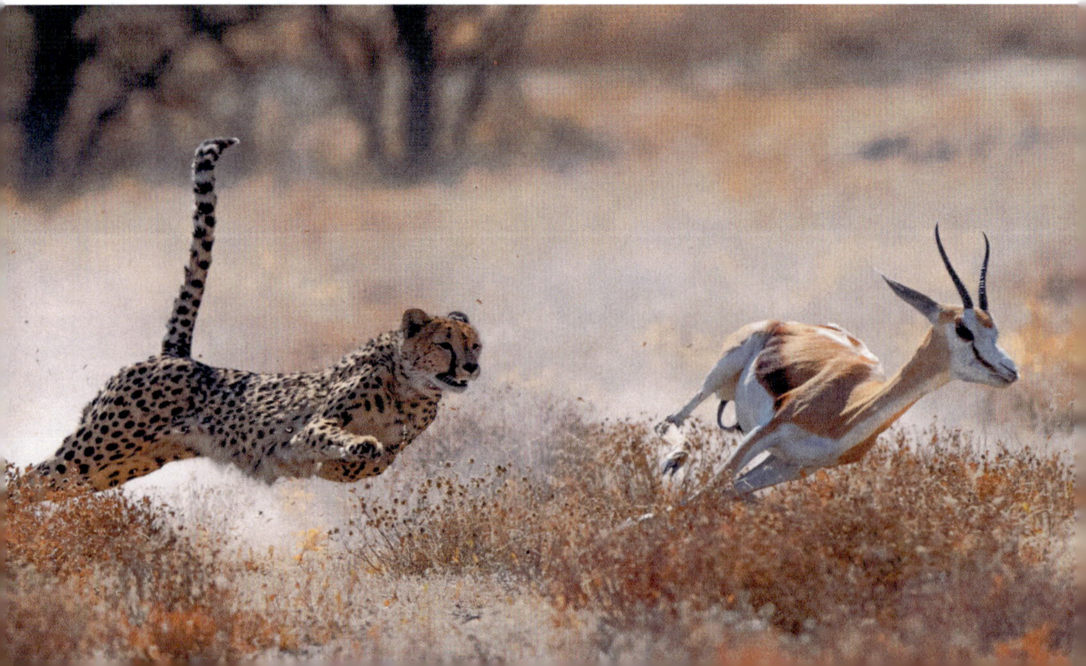

However, if the strong are careless or ignorant, they may not survive as illustrated in the picture below:

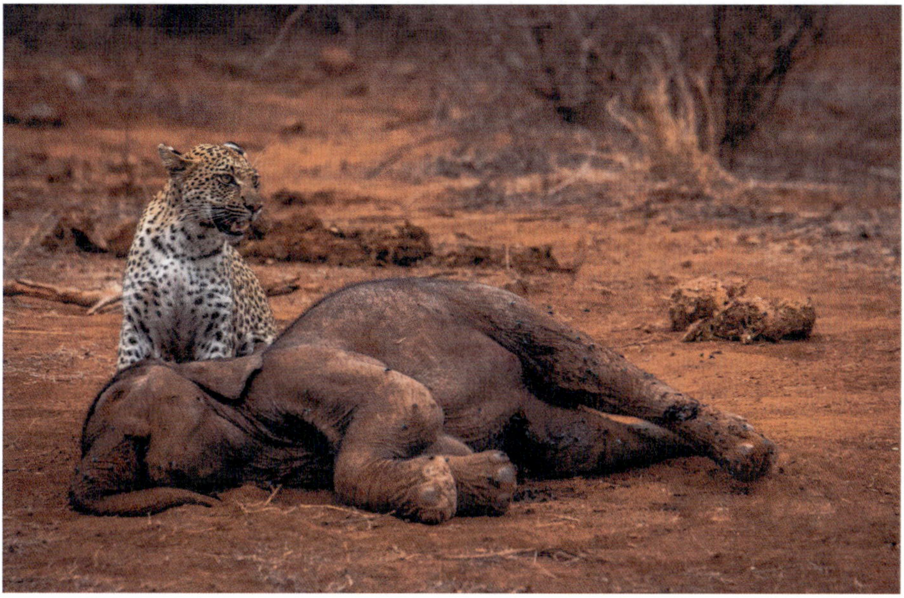

Survival doesn't depend on strength alone. It also requires intelligence or instinct, i.e., cautiousness, cruelty, and selfishness. Animals that don't have enough of these traits will not survive.

Likewise, human society is full of dangers and cruelty so humans depend on these traits to survive. That is, humans have to be cautious, cruel, and selfish. But humans are smarter than other kinds of animals, these traits are not only a means of survival but a tool to seek wealth, fame, and honor. Some people may possess too much of these traits to the point where they become greedy, selfish, cruel, and vengeful — the dark sides of humans. They can do anything for themselves without thinking about how others may suffer. There are so many of these people in our society.

Thus, overly innocent people may not survive this cruel and selfish society. For example, when young children become adults and have to live in the outside world on their own, Nature gives them these instincts or traits for survival when they start to become teenagers, the age with a number of physical and psychological changes. In terms of the psychological changes, young and gentle children will turn into teenagers who are cautious, cruel, and selfish in order for them to survive. The kind of love that they have toward their parents changes as well. It will not be as innocent as before because it has been affected by the natural traits that I described earlier.

The parents can often recognize these changes. They can tell that their children have grown into teenagers from the character change, for example, from being soft and gentle to stubborn, aggressive, and disobedient. Although children seem to change in a negative way, it's necessary for their survival and Nature must make this happen. And no matter how much their emotions and behaviors change, their real selves remain the same. That is, "they still love their parents more than anyone else."

Pure love of children and the limitation of natural law

When God or Nature created stars and planets including the Earth and the Sun. At the time, if gravity had not been created, each of these stars and planets would have its own orbit and the solar system would not exist. That is, the Sun wouldn't be the center of the universe. There would be neither seasons nor daytime and nighttime on Earth. The temperature would be so low that no animals could survive.

But Nature builds gravity. As a result, the Earth orbits the Sun. The force created was so "well-designed" it brings about different kinds of balance on Earth such as

- Balance to the environment: There are rain, streams, rivers, and fresh air.
- Balance to the ecosystem: Animals and plants mutually benefit from each other to the point where they can sustain their species for hundreds of thousand years.

Plants and animals exist due to the gravity of the Earth. Although this force has a tremendous influence, humans don't feel that way. This kind of balance has been going on for ages. We tend to take it for granted and think that "that's just the way it is" without realizing that the balance is caused by gravity or certain kinds of force. For example, we see the falling rain, fruits falling from the trees, or children sliding down a slider as something normal. We don't feel that there must be a mechanism behind these phenomena until Sir Isaac Newton, the great mathematician, saw an apple falling from a tree and was curious why it was falling from top to bottom. Eventually, he discovered that gravity caused the apple to fall to the ground. Furthermore, gravity is the reason the moon revolves around the Earth. Without this force, the moon would keep floating straight pass the Earth.

Similarly, for humans to live together as a society, Nature also builds a kind of force that will attract them to be together. Without this force, they won't get together for a long time because they would want to "separate," to walk on their own paths the same way the moon would find its own route if the Earth's gravity stopped functioning. Therefore, Nature created a kind of force called "love" to ensure that humans will remain together. Love is always on standby to bring them happiness so they prefer living together than staying alone as before. In fact, they would like to be together as long as possible. This is how human society originated. The smallest unit is "a family." When there are more and more families, a community or a country is founded.

Love created by Nature was so "well-designed" it has brought not only happiness but a number of favorable consequences. These consequences enrich family lives in many ways, for example,

- Bringing the loveliest children to their parents.
- Making a connection between parents and children as if they were 2 smartphones linked together via Bluetooth. Once children have certain feelings, their parents can sense those feelings instantly. It's no surprise that "when children are feeling joy," the parents become joyful as well.
- Creating the funniest comedians in the world right at home: This turns the "duty" of raising children into "fun activities" because taking care of children often brings smiles and laughter to their parents.

Love and its consequences are important mechanisms behind the development of family lives and human society in pretty much the same way as gravity is behind different natural phenomena like an apple falling from a tree. But we're so familiar with these things (human society and natural phenomena), we think they just occur by themselves and no mechanisms are playing their roles behind the scenes. We take these mechanisms for granted and don't give them any credits.

Being unable to see the value of "gravity" may not affect our lives that much. But failing to see the value of "love" can definitely affect our lives as seen in the case study. Because when we cannot see how important love is, our hearts become empty and we will seek other things to fill the emptiness. Focusing on searching for material things that help fulfill our lives will further minimize the importance of love. In addition, certain situations could lessen the value of love, for example, stress from financial situations (running short of money, or heavily in debt) and being addicted to alcohol, gambling, drugs, or even smartphones. People who don't value love or those in the abovementioned situations are likely to bring violence to their families, e.g., engaging in physical abuse, fighting, and abandoning their lovers.

Thus, the natural law that "love will connect humans through happiness it brings." may not always be true. Mechanisms of love do have a limitation: "Although God or Nature can build wonderful laws for humans, God or Nature cannot force the outcomes to always go as planned." Humans also need to take care of themselves and the love they have so these mechanisms can function at full capacity. That is, to bring happiness to humans' lives.

Married Couples with Children and Positive Changes

Not only does having children help parents discover true and pure love but it also brings about important psychological changes. Some of them are listed below.

Thoughts and behaviors

Each human being has unique thoughts and behaviors of their own. We call these thoughts and behaviors "habits," which can change. But it is unlikely to be successful. Habits of a person tend to stay the same for the rest of their life.

- Some people are narrow-minded or never forgive anyone.
- Some people look stressful all the time and never chitchat, laugh, or smile.

- Some people think only about their own benefits and never give away anything to anyone.
- Some people never accept that they make mistakes and often blame someone else for their own mistakes.

Each person has both good and bad habits (in certain matters). Our habits, whether good or bad, are based on several factors such as genes, genders, emotions, family background, upbringing, parents' trait values, religions, and cultures.

Habits indicate not only a person's behaviors and expression but what will happen to them in the future, for instance:

- People who are not discouraged and stay patient can complete their assignments successfully, which helps them progress in their careers.
- Those who are always cheerful and think positively can easily find happiness in their lives either at work or in their personal lives. Being happy means good mental health, which will lead to good physical health and long lives.

Since habits are very important because they affect our future, if our habits change, our future will change as well. Although habits are hard to change, when a married couple has a child, the new environment may affect their behaviors and habits. For example,

- When the child is still an infant, the parents have to look after it very closely or 24 hours per day. Daily activities that they have to do include changing diapers, cleaning the baby's bottom, mixing the formula, feeding it, carrying the infant while walking around, and getting the baby to go to sleep. The parents have to go through these activities several times per day for at least a year. So, parents look very exhausted due to a lack of sleep. But this also trains them to be patient and willing to make sacrifices.
- When the child starts to grow, the parents have to teach their child about almost everything, such as using a spoon and a glass, eating, sitting, and walking. The child is likely to be disobedient or cannot follow the parents' instructions, e.g., making a mess while eating, breaking things, throwing up on the parents, tripping or falling down the stairs and bumping his/her head. Experienced parents will be able to solve problems instantly. Once a problem is solved, they will continue teaching the child as if nothing had happened. They will not overreact by yelling at or punishing the kid unreasonably, knowing that doing so will worsen the situation. So, this trains the parents to be calm and to forgive.
- Generally, parents usually buy toys for the kids to make them happy and try to spend time with them. Thus, there are a lot of toys and laughter in these families. Parents also take the kids to amusement parks, zoos, shopping malls, or snow towns to entertain them and let them learn about things in the outside world. Spending time with children, playing with them, and visiting places for children are "the key" to soften adults' hearts. These parents usually forget about their stress. They'll play and laugh as though they were little kids once again. This turns the parents into joyful and relaxing people.

"Raising a child" takes more than ten years. What I've described will happen again and again throughout those years. The parents' behaviors I mentioned will be repeated numerous times. Having to do what they've never done before a number of times eventually forms "new habits." Willingness to sacrifice, patience, forgiveness, and calmness are all good habits because they help us lead our lives more efficiently and smoothly. Therefore, having children is an important turning point that allows the parents to prepare themselves to take better care of their families and to lead everyone including themselves to better destinations in their lives.

Childhood's Unanswered Questions

When we were young, we all had questions or doubts in our minds, for instance:

- Why doesn't my mother love me?
- Why does my mother keep spanking me?
- Why do my mom and dad fight all the time?
- Why doesn't my mother buy me toys?
- Why does my mom love my younger brother/sister more than me?
- Why does my mom make me brush my teeth?

- Why aren't we as rich as others? (Why don't we have things that others do?)
- Why does my mother make me go to school and do homework?

Even when we've grown up into adults, these questions still linger in our subconscious along with disappointment and sadness about those events. And even though more than a decade has passed, many people still remember these matters. There are still a large number of people who're suffering from past events. For example,

- painful feeling due to the love from their mothers being taken away by his/her siblings
- feeling depressed from seeing their parents fighting
- feeling frustrated from being spanked or punished without having done anything wrong
- disappointment from not getting what they want, e.g., toys, smartphones, and trips with friends

These unanswered questions and the pain that follows are fixed in their subconscious and negatively affect their mental health. Solving these hidden unanswered questions can heal these wounds in their hearts so that they will no longer suffer from the pain in the past. I'll use the following case to explain how "having children" can help solve these unanswered questions.

Malee and the Scar on Her Right Arm

Malee is a good-looking nurse from upcountry. She came to Bangkok for her studies and continue to work there after graduation. Growing up in a poor family, she knows the value of money. She works hard and spends her money wisely so she could save enough money to send home to her mother every month. Therefore, she doesn't have financial problems. However, one thing that she's suffering from is "the scar on her right arm." This scar was caused by hot water spilled on her arm when she was 7. It runs from her wrist to her elbow or almost the length of her arm.

Although the scar itself doesn't cause any pain, beauty is quite important for women. Having a big scar with almost the length of her arm is hurtful for Malee. She hates this scar. What's more, it affects her work because whenever she's measuring patients' blood pressure or drawing patients' blood for a test, some patients look at the scar with fear or in disgust. Thus, she usually wears a long-sleeved shirt so that no one can see it and she'll forget about it for a while.

But in any case, her mind is usually wandering around this scar even though decades have gone by. She knows that accidents can be avoided. "If my mother had been more careful, I wouldn't have been injured by the hot water." She's still so angry with her mother for letting this happened to her. She has never gone back to visit her mother since she graduated. But she still sends her money along with an excuse that she's busy and often has to be on duty.

After working at the hospital for 2 years, she got married and her family life is running smoothly. She has one child called "Nalin," a very restless girl, runs around all day. With her scar in mind, Malee has been keeping a close eye on her child. When it's necessary to go out, she would hire someone to look after Nalin. She believes that "Accidents can be avoided and history must not repeat itself. Nalin must not have a serious accident."

No matter how cautious she has been, Nalin still has an accident occasionally, e.g., a chin injury, a torn gum, a torn-off nail, and a scratch. The worst case was when a dice slipped down her throat when she was 3 years old. Malee can still remember that event very well. On that day, Nalin was playing the Monopoly game her mom just bought her. In the package, there was a dice and a tube-shaped cup for throwing the dice. Malee was watching TV nearby while Nalin was playing the game. At one point, Nalin pretended that she was going to take a sip from the cup, forgetting that there was a dice in there. As a result, the dice fell down her throat and she was too young to spit it out. The dice went through her throat to her stomach instantly. Nalin yelled out loudly "Mom! ... Mom, the dice fell down my throat!" Malee was shocked. She took her daughter to see a doctor in a hurry. The doctor told her to look for the dice in Nalin's feces every day because there was a good chance it would come out by itself. He also told her that if it did not come out and her daughter happened to have a stomachache, he would consider giving Nalin surgery.

After 2 days, the dice still didn't come out. Malee was stressed. She was afraid that her daughter would have to undergo an operation. She had been very nervous since the beginning of the incident. And, at last, on the 3rd day, she found the dice in her child's feces. She yelled out with joy, "I found it! I found it!"

This incident made her recall the day hot water spilled on her and realized that when a child had an injury, the person who suffered the most was the mother. Although Nalin had not gone through an operation and didn't even bleed, Malee was still so stressed out. What if hot water had been spilled on Nalin's arm instead, how stressful it would have been for her? When she reflected on the past accidents that happened to Nalin, she realized that she was always there during those accidents. So, she was never negligent. But the accidents happened so fast it was impossible to prevent them in time. At that exact moment, the hatred toward her mother has turned into sympathy.

After she has come to realize this, she starts to feel that the scar on her arm is no longer hurtful. She doesn't pay attention to the scar anymore. After 2 weeks passed by, Malee, her husband, and her daughter went to visit Malee's mother in her hometown. Everyone was happy and had a good time talking to each other.

When people live together, one thing that cannot be avoided is a dispute, which is not surprising at all because "your tongue and your teeth" were particularly well designed to work together but they still get in each other's way sometimes. Conflicts in a family are normal. These conflicts can be eased when both sides understand each other. And they would understand even more deeply if they had switched their roles. For example, the tongue has to function as the teeth or the teeth have to work as the tongue. Therefore, when Malee has become a mother, she started to understand those past events. This understanding completely wiped out anger in her subconscious. Moreover, the unanswered questions such as "Why did my mom always spank me?" and "Why did my mom and dad keep fighting?" can finally be answered as well when one becomes a mother.

"Having children" not only solves problems from the past, but it can improve the relationship of family members. A large number of families are suffering from problems dealing with "young love." But when they have children, "true or pure love" from their children will enter these parents' lives. And this kind of love can heal all wounds or replace the "young love" that they have lost.

Conclusions: The Roles of This Book and What Readers May Gain From it

This book plays
4 important roles:

1. As a brochure for Nature's work

There are a large number of entertainment products. These products are advertised in numerous ways. One way is by using brochures to advertise what good things these products can offer and why we should buy them. For example, how are the new models of smartphones better than the previous ones? How is this new condo worth your money? And how gorgeous will you look if you use this set of cosmetics? But we never have a brochure offering an explanation about family lives with children although it is essential for us. Explanations for family lives are like a brochure describing the advantages of building a family and this will help Nature's works stand out even among entertainment products advertised in various forms. Learning about facts in this book will also help readers make smart choices in their lives. They will be aware of knowledge from those who have chosen to build their families. This knowledge consists of overlooked facts because no one has explained them in such great detail.

2. As the user's manual for parents with children

This book describes family matters scientifically, therefore, the readers should be able to understand them deeply. Such an understanding will help them lead better family lives because doubts in their minds have been answered logically. They can be confident that the answers to these questions are accurate:

- Why does raising a child have to be troublesome, exhausting, and long-lasting?
- Although taking care of a child is exhausting, why do parents enjoy their lives more than before?
- Why do children become disobedient when they turn into teenagers?

This understanding will help your family life continue more smoothly. The contents of this book range from fundamental matters to small details. Therefore, reading this book should help you succeed in leading your family life.

3. As a means of returning fairness to children

God or Nature builds family life in a way that allows family members to be mutually supportive. That is, parents support their children by taking care of them and offering them security and education whereas children support their parents by

- providing a source of happiness in the families and helping parents see their life goals more clearly.
- bringing positive changes to their parents' habits, e.g., becoming more responsible, more willing to make sacrifices, and more mature. These new habits improve parents' lives.
- becoming caregivers when their parents grow old or cannot help themselves.

However, these roles of children tend to be abstract or hard to see. People always think that only the parents take on the role of givers. But in reality, children also play an important role in helping their parents succeed. This book not only returns fairness to children but also helps us understand the kind of love in their hearts.

Humans know that love is a source of happiness so they struggle to find love in their lives. Nevertheless, true love or pure love is hard to find. They are likely to end up with deception and untrue love from people who try to take advantage of them. Some people cannot find true or pure love even when they turn old. They feel that "something is missing in their lives" and continue to search for their true love.

It's rather surprising that although true love or pure love is hard to find, it can be found quite easily in the hearts of all children. This kind of love from children not only brings happiness but is the key to filling "the missing part" in adults' hearts.

4. As a new aspect of physics

If you look carefully, you'll see that things that Nature has created change endlessly. These changes are in the form of the cycle that repeats itself over and over again unceasingly. For example,

- Water keeps evaporating, turns into the rain, and returns to the surface of the Earth. Then, the rain continues to evaporate.
- Oxygen in the air is used all the time, but the Earth never runs out of it because plants keep producing new oxygen to replace it.
- The Earth never stops revolving around the Sun. When one round ends, another begins. This has been going on for a long time.

These phenomena carry on uninterrupted for many million years because Nature has mechanisms to keep the processes running one after another in balance. Without these natural laws to control them, these processes would have ceased to exist a long time ago. Some of the mechanisms that control these phenomena are listed below:

- The Laws of Evaporation and Condensation cause the rain to fall on the surface of the Earth.
- The Law of Biochemistry causes photosynthesis. Due to this law, plants can generate oxygen for the Earth.
- The Law of Gravity keeps the orbit of the stars and planets stable and in balance.

Humans know about these laws quite well from the subject called "Physics" (from the Greek root "phusikos" meaning "about nature") they learned in school. The meaning of the word "nature" is very wide. Physics is divided into various branches, e.g., astrophysics, biophysics, geophysics, and chemical physics.

In the same vein, to sustain human species, Nature creates laws or mechanisms to control their ways of living so that they build warm families. As long as families survive, human society will continue to exist because families are a foundation of society. Some examples of natural mechanisms are:

- Offering intense and passionate love for young couples to initiate other processes that will follow.
- Creating the loveliest children in the world, the funniest comedians in the world, and a connection between parents and children to ensure that all processes will bring happiness to everyone involved.
- Giving true and pure love to fill the parents' hearts to prevent troubles and exhaustion from bothering them psychologically.
- Offering caregivers who will take good care of their parents to reward those parents who made sacrifices for their families.

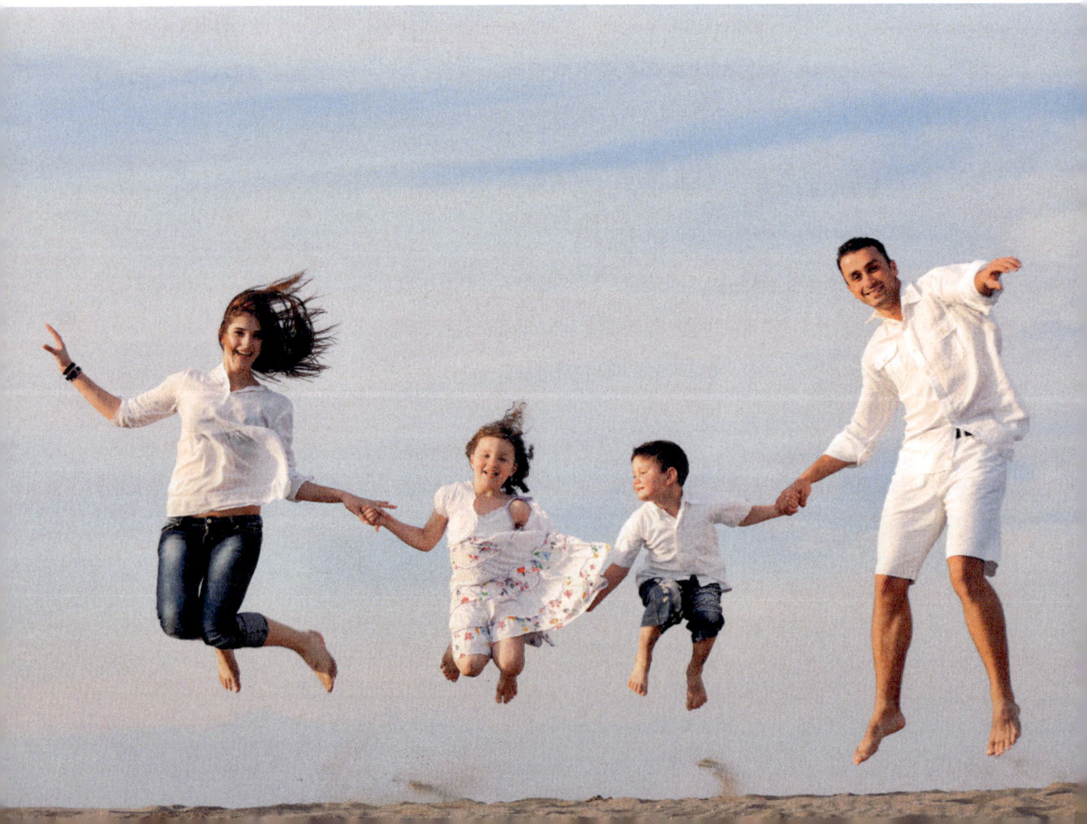

These mechanisms have been helping family lives go on in cycles until these days. Since the mechanisms I mentioned in this book were created by Nature, they can also be categorized as the laws of physics. Physics is not limited to a mass of things, energy, or stars and planets but also deals with emotions and feelings. To facilitate reference, I'll call these laws "Psychophysics" which are mechanisms behind the creation of human society and family lives. (The word "Psychophysics" has already been used before with a different definition or to describe an aspect different from the one mentioned in this book.)

Different branches of Physics that we have learned about such as Astrophysics, Biophysics, and Chemical physics help educate us so that we have a better understanding of nature and live with nature in harmony. While an understanding of Psychophysics helps us understand our own minds, emotions and feelings. This kind of understanding is crucial because it will assist us in making better choices about our ways of living. That is the main goal of this book.

The content of this book is rather complicated and different from what you've heard before.

Reading this book several times will help you understand it better and will make the book more valuable because what you learn from it **will increase tremendously,** making it worth your money.

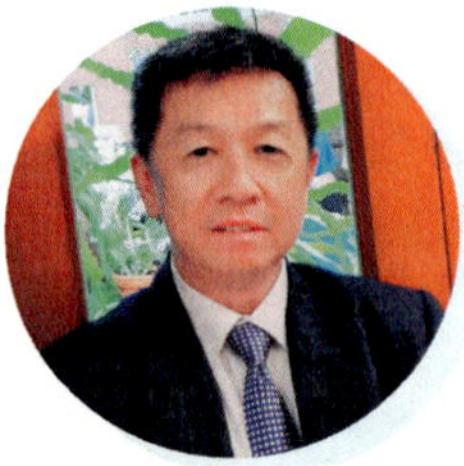

Contact Information:

kasemkasem007

korbsrisate@gmail.com

https://www.facebook.com/kasemkorbsrisate

About the Author

Kasem Korbsrisate, M.D.

Born: April 1962

Education

Kindergarten and junior elementary school:
Pornprasartwittaya School, Taladplu, Thonburi

Senior elementary school:
Sitwattana School, Bangkok Noi, Bangkok

Junior high school:
Suwannaramwittayakom School, Bangkok Noi, Bangkok

Senior high school:
Triam Udom Suksa School

University: (1979 – 1984)
Faculty of Medicine, Ramathibodi Hospital

Specialist: (1988 – 1990)
Otolaryngology, Faculty of Medicine, Chiang Mai University

Work experiences:

1985 – 1987: Intern
Department of MTB, Yotse Lung Disease Center

1991 – 1996:
Ear, nose, and throat doctor
Taksin Hospital

1996 – 2016:
Ear, nose, and throat doctor
Kasemrad Hospital, Bang Khae

2009 – Present:
Ear, nose, and throat doctor
Eye Ear Nose Throat Hospital

Family

Married with 3 children

Made in United States
Orlando, FL
04 November 2026

90201768R00093